护 理 专 业 医 教 协 同 创 新 教 材
德技并修/课证融通/融媒体/新形态教材

总主编　杜天信　胡仕坤

供高职高专护理学、助产学类专业用

护理心理学
Nursing Psychology

主编　骆焕丽　汪玉兰

英汉对照

U0340322

郑州大学出版社

图书在版编目(CIP)数据

护理心理学：英汉对照 / 骆焕丽，汪玉兰主编. -- 郑州：郑州大学出版社，2023. 6
护理专业医教协同创新教材
ISBN 978-7-5645-9501-2

Ⅰ.①护…　Ⅱ.①骆…②汪…　Ⅲ.①护理学 - 医学心理学 - 教材 - 英、汉　Ⅳ.①R471

中国国家版本馆 CIP 数据核字(2023)第 029696 号

护理心理学

HULI XINLIXUE

策划编辑	陈文静		封面设计	苏永生
责任编辑	吕笑娟		版式设计	苏永生
责任校对	张　楠		责任监制	李瑞卿

出版发行	郑州大学出版社		地　　址	郑州市大学路 40 号(450052)
出 版 人	孙保营		网　　址	http://www.zzup.cn
经　　销	全国新华书店		发行电话	0371-66966070
印　　刷	郑州宁昌印务有限公司			
开　　本	850 mm×1 168 mm　1 / 16			
印　　张	15		字　　数	503 千字
版　　次	2023 年 6 月第 1 版		印　　次	2023 年 6 月第 1 次印刷

书　　号	ISBN 978-7-5645-9501-2		定　　价	46.50 元

河南护理职业学院院级教育教学改革研究与实践项目：中外合作办学《护理心理学》课程双语教材的开发研究（项目编号 HHJG-2022-YB27）

作者名单

主　编　骆焕丽　汪玉兰

副主编　戴　路

编　者（以姓氏笔画为序）

王红如（河南护理职业学院）

苏艳梅（河南护理职业学院）

汪玉兰（河南护理职业学院）

陈　品（濮阳市安阳地区医院）

陈　晶（河南护理职业学院）

赵露露（河南护理职业学院）

娄安琪（河南护理职业学院）

骆焕丽（河南护理职业学院）

靳晓霞（河南护理职业学院）

戴　路（河南护理职业学院）

前　言

近年来,为认真落实河南省《关于做好新时期教育对外开放工作的实施意见》,服务"一带一路"建设,进一步扩大对外合作交流,高校需培养具有国际视野和国际竞争力的高水平护理人才。

教材是课程的重要载体和教学方法选择的基础,也是实现人才培养目的的必备工具。习近平总书记在二十大报告中指出,推进健康中国建设。坚持人民至上、生命至上,推动构建人类卫生健康共同体。因此,本教材在编写过程中,以护理人才基本能力培养为本位,依据学习者的认知结构,结合中外护理工作岗位任务和工作过程对护理人员在"认知、情感、态度和技能"方面的实际需要,重在培养护理人员的专业素养,并通过内容创新与医教协同,多角度渗透人文素养和创新思维等理念。

本教材共二十一章,分别为护理心理学概述、发展心理学概述、婴儿的发展、幼儿的发展、学龄前期儿童的发展、学龄期儿童的发展、青少年的发展、成年早中期个体的发展、成年晚期个体的发展、学习、智力、动机、情绪、记忆、人格、疾病、残疾、住院治疗、损失和哀伤、临终护理及压力管理。在内容上,本教材以学生够用为基本原则,重在通俗易懂、简明扼要,将心理学的基本观点和技能体现在教材中,便于学生理解、掌握,是护理心理学的入门教材。在结构上,本教材兼顾理论和实践应用的需要,更新了护理心理学体系结构,赋予本学科知识体系以崭新的构架,加强理论性,注重实践性,体现逻辑性。

教材各章编写安排如下:英文部分 Chapter 1 由骆焕丽撰写,Chapter 2 至 Chapter 8、Chapter 11、Chapter 17、Chapter 18、Chapter 20 由汪玉兰撰写,Chapter 9 由赵露露撰写,Chapter 10、Chapter 15、Chapter 19 由戴路撰写,Chapter 12 至 Chapter 14 由苏艳梅撰写,Chapter 16 由王红如撰写,Chapter 21 由靳晓霞撰写。中文部分第一章、第十七章由汪玉兰撰写,第二章至第九章由娄安琪撰写,第十章、第十五章、第十九章由戴路撰写,第十一章、第十八章第二节第三节、第二十章由陈晶撰写,第十八章第一节由陈品撰写,第十二章至第十四章由苏艳梅撰写,第十六章由王红如撰写,第二十一章由靳晓霞撰写。

在教材的编写过程中,编者力求并坚持将我国护理心理学教育国际化和特色化目标较好地整合体现在教材中。本教材虽为中外合作办学所用的双语教材,但由于它体现了国际护理心理学教育的新理念和双语编写的特色,所以也适用于所有护理专业学生和有志于从事国际护理工作的护理人员。

本书的编者均具有"双师型"教师资质,但由于编者知识的限制,书中也难免会有不尽如人意之处,真诚希望广大读者提出宝贵意见,以便再版时加以修订,使之日臻完善。

编 者

2023 年 4 月

目 录

Chapter 1　Overview of Nursing Psychology ·· 001

　　Section 1　Introduction to Nursing Psychology ·· 001

　　　　1.1.1　Concept of psychology ··· 001

　　　　1.1.2　Concept of nursing psychology ·· 001

　　　　1.1.3　Significance of nursing psychology ·· 001

　　　　1.1.4　Research tasks of nursing psychology ······································ 002

　　Section 2　Important Theories of Psychology ··· 003

　　　　1.2.1　Psychodynamic theory ··· 003

　　　　1.2.2　Behaviorism theory ··· 004

　　　　1.2.3　Humanistic theory ·· 005

　　　　1.2.4　Cognitive theory ··· 005

Chapter 2　Overview of Developmental Psychology ····································· 007

　　Section 1　Overview of Developmental Psychology Research ······················ 007

　　　　2.1.1　Growth ··· 007

　　　　2.1.2　Development ·· 007

　　　　2.1.3　Stage of individual development ·· 007

　　Section 2　Principle Factors and Influencing Factors of Individual Growth and Development

　　　　·· 009

　　　　2.2.1　Principle of development ··· 009

　　　　2.2.2　Factors that affect individual development ································· 010

　　　　2.2.3　Factors affecting individual growth and development ······················ 010

Chapter 3　Development of Infants ·· 012

　　Section 1　Physiological Development of Infants ······································ 012

　　　　3.1.1　Body development of infants ··· 012

　　　　3.1.2　Motor development of infants ·· 013

　　Section 2　Cognitive Development of Infants ·· 014

　　　　3.2.1　Development of perception ··· 014

    3.2.2   Development of attention ·· 015

   Section 3   Infant Emotional and Social Development ························· 015

    3.3.1   Emotional development ··· 015

    3.3.2   Socialization of infant emotions ·································· 015

   Section 4   Nursing Care of Babies ·· 015

    3.4.1   Satisfy sucking needs ··· 016

    3.4.2   Establish eating habits ·· 016

    3.4.3   Don't begrudge your hugs ·· 016

Chapter 4   Development of Young Children ··································· 017

   Section 1   Physiological and Cognitive Development of Young Children ······· 017

    4.1.1   Physical development of young children ······················ 017

    4.1.2   Cognitive development of young children ····················· 017

   Section 2   Emotional and Personality Development in Early Childhood ······· 018

    4.2.1   Parents' emotional support ··· 018

    4.2.2   Attachment behavior and separation anxiety ················· 019

    4.2.3   Children's sense of independence ······························· 019

   Section 3   Health Care for Young Children ······································ 019

    4.3.1   Physical care ·· 020

    4.3.2   Social capability care ··· 020

    4.3.3   Psychological care ·· 020

Chapter 5   Development of Preschool Children ································ 022

   Section 1   Physiological Development of Preschool Children ··············· 022

    5.1.1   Body development ·· 022

    5.1.2   Brain development ·· 022

    5.1.3   Sports development ··· 023

   Section 2   Cognitive Development of Preschool Children ·················· 023

    5.2.1   Development of language ·· 023

    5.2.2   Characteristics of attention development ······················ 023

    5.2.3   Characteristics of imagination development ··················· 024

    5.2.4   Development of thinking ··· 024

   Section 3   Psychological Development of Preschool Children ·············· 024

    5.3.1   Active conflict with guilt ·· 024

    5.3.2   Development of self-awareness ···································· 024

   Section 4   Emotional Development of Preschool Children ·················· 025

    5.4.1   Rapid development of empathy ···································· 025

    5.4.2　Emotional understanding depends on social knowledge ················· 025

  Section 5　Health Assessment and Nursing of Preschool Children ················· 026

    5.5.1　Nutrition ················· 026

    5.5.2　Daily activities ················· 026

    5.5.3　To protect the teeth ················· 027

Chapter 6　Development of School-age Children ················· 028

  Section 1　Physiological Development of School-age Children ················· 028

  Section 2　Elementary School-age Children's Psychological Development ················· 029

    6.2.1　Conflict of diligence and inferiority ················· 029

    6.2.2　Cognitive development of school-age children ················· 030

  Section 3　Elementary School-age Children's Emotional and Personality Development ········· 031

    6.3.1　Emotional development of school-age children ················· 031

    6.3.2　Character development of school-age children ················· 031

  Section 4　Physical and Mental Care of School-age Children ················· 032

    6.4.1　Physical care work ················· 032

    6.4.2　Psychological care work ················· 032

Chapter 7　Development of Adolescents ················· 034

  Section 1　Physiological Development of Adolescent ················· 034

    7.1.1　Changes in body shape ················· 034

    7.1.2　Enhancement of body functions ················· 035

    7.1.3　Sexual development and maturation ················· 036

  Section 2　Psychological Development of Adolescent ················· 036

    7.2.1　Development of self-awareness ················· 037

    7.2.2　Characteristics of emotional development ················· 038

    7.2.3　Characteristics of interpersonal communication ················· 038

  Section 3　Cognitive Development of Adolescent ················· 039

  Section 4　Physical and Mental Care of Adolescent ················· 040

    7.4.1　Psychological care ················· 040

    7.4.2　Physical health care ················· 040

Chapter 8　Development of Individuals in Early and Middle Adulthood ················· 042

  Section 1　Overview for Individual in Early Adulthood ················· 042

    8.1.1　Age limit for early adulthood ················· 042

    8.1.2　General characteristics of early adulthood ················· 042

    8.1.3　Cognitive characteristics of early adulthood ················· 043

  Section 2　Overview for Individual in Middle Adulthood ················· 044

Section 3　Individual Care and Wellness Planning for Early and Middle Adulthood　·········· 044

　　8.3.1　Individual psychological care ··· 044

　　8.3.2　Individual body care ··· 045

Chapter 9　Development of Individuals in Late Adulthood　······································ 047

　Section 1　Cognitive Characteristics of Late Adulthood　······························· 047

　　9.1.1　Significant degenerative changes in perception　······························· 047

　　9.1.2　Memory declines with age　·· 048

　　9.1.3　Changes in thinking　·· 048

　Section 2　Emotional Characteristics in Late Adulthood ································· 048

　　9.2.1　It is easier to have negative emotions　·· 049

　　9.2.2　Deep and lasting emotional experience　··· 049

　Section 3　Nursing Work in Late Adulthood　··· 049

　　9.3.1　Common health problems in late adulthood　······························· 050

　　9.3.2　Nursing and health care measures in late adulthood ····················· 050

Chapter 10　Learning　··· 052

　Section 1　Concept of Learning　··· 052

　　10.1.1　Definition of learning　·· 052

　　10.1.2　Learning of newborns　·· 052

　Section 2　Learning Theories in the Early Stage　······························· 053

　　10.2.1　Classical conditioning　·· 053

　　10.2.2　Operant conditioning ··· 055

　　10.2.3　Social learning theory　·· 058

Chapter 11　Intelligence　··· 060

　Section 1　Overview of Intelligence　··· 060

　　11.1.1　Intelligence theory　·· 060

　　11.1.2　Multiple intelligences theory ··· 060

　Section 2　Intelligence and IQ　··· 062

　　11.2.1　Intelligence test　··· 062

　　11.2.2　Other tests ·· 062

　　11.2.3　Because of factors affecting intelligence　····························· 062

　Section 3　Emotional Quotient　··· 064

Chapter 12　Motivation　··· 065

　Section 1　General Concepts of Motivation　··· 065

　　12.1.1　Motivated behaviour　··· 065

　　12.1.2　A model of motivation　·· 065

4

Section 2　Types of Motives and Related Theories ……………………………………… 066

　12.2.1　Types of motives ……………………………………………………………… 066

　12.2.2　Humanistic theory …………………………………………………………… 067

Section 3　Application in Clinical Nursing ……………………………………………… 069

　12.3.1　Application of needs in clinical nursing ………………………………………… 069

　12.3.2　Application of motivation in clinical nursing …………………………………… 069

Chapter 13　Emotion ……………………………………………………………………… 070

Section 1　Concept and Elements of Emotion …………………………………………… 070

　13.1.1　Concept of emotion …………………………………………………………… 070

　13.1.2　Elements of emotion …………………………………………………………… 070

Section 2　Emotional Development and Influencing Factors …………………………… 071

　13.2.1　Emotional development ………………………………………………………… 071

　13.2.2　Factors that affect emotional development …………………………………… 072

Chapter 14　Memory ……………………………………………………………………… 073

Section 1　Concept and Types of Memory ……………………………………………… 073

　14.1.1　Concept of memory …………………………………………………………… 073

　14.1.2　Types of memory ……………………………………………………………… 074

Section 2　Forgetting ……………………………………………………………………… 075

　14.2.1　Process of forgetting …………………………………………………………… 075

　14.2.2　Cause of forgetting …………………………………………………………… 076

Chapter 15　Personality …………………………………………………………………… 077

Section 1　Definition and Significance of Personality …………………………………… 077

　15.1.1　Definition ……………………………………………………………………… 077

　15.1.2　Purpose of studying personality ………………………………………………… 077

Section 2　Development of Personality …………………………………………………… 078

　15.2.1　Three aspects of personality according to behavierist ………………………… 078

　15.2.2　Psychoanalytic approach ……………………………………………………… 078

　15.2.3　Humanistic approach …………………………………………………………… 080

Chapter 16　Disease ……………………………………………………………………… 082

Section 1　Overview ……………………………………………………………………… 082

　16.1.1　Basic concepts ………………………………………………………………… 082

　16.1.2　Classification of diseases ……………………………………………………… 083

　16.1.3　The factor that affect the disease ……………………………………………… 083

　16.1.4　The stage of the disease ……………………………………………………… 084

　16.1.5　The impact of the disease on patients,families and society ………………… 085

Section 2 Roles of Patiens and Nurses ················· 086

    16.2.1 Role of the patient ················· 086

    16.2.2 Psychological reactions of patients with malignant tumors ················· 088

    16.2.3 The role of nurses ················· 089

Chapter 17 Disability ················· 090

Section 1 Overview ················· 090

    17.1.1 Concept of disability ················· 090

    17.1.2 Caregivers learn the meaning of disability ················· 090

    17.1.3 Classification of disability ················· 090

    17.1.4 Causes of disabilities ················· 091

Section 2 Mental Response of the Disabled ················· 091

Chapter 18 Hospitalization ················· 093

Section 1 Overview ················· 093

    18.1.1 Concept of hospitalization ················· 093

    18.1.2 Psychological nursing procedures ················· 093

Section 2 Psychological Characteristics of Hospitalized Patients at Different Ages ················· 094

    18.2.1 Psychological characteristics of children patients ················· 094

    18.2.2 Psychological characteristics of young patients ················· 094

    18.2.3 Psychological characteristics of middle-aged patients ················· 095

    18.2.4 Psychological characteristics of elderly patients ················· 096

Section 3 Emotional Problems of Psychological Nursing ················· 096

    18.3.1 Anxiety ················· 097

    18.3.2 Depression ················· 097

    18.3.3 Fear ················· 098

    18.3.4 Anger ················· 098

Chapter 19 Loss and Grief ················· 099

Section 1 Loss ················· 099

    19.1.1 Definition of loss ················· 099

    19.1.2 Type of loss ················· 100

Section 2 Grief ················· 100

    19.2.1 Definition of grief ················· 100

    19.2.2 Types of grief ················· 101

    19.2.3 Stages of grieving ················· 101

    19.2.4 Assisting the grieving persons ················· 102

Section 3　　Lose and Greif in Medical Condition ·· 103

　　19.3.1　Communicating with dying adult patients ·································· 103

　　19.3.2　Communicating with dying child patients ·································· 103

　　19.3.3　Death in accdent and emergency departments ·························· 104

Chapter 20　End-of-life Care ·· 106

　Section 1　　Near Death and Dying ·· 106

　　20.1.1　Concept ··· 106

　　20.1.2　Death standard ·· 106

　　20.1.3　Stages of the death process ·· 107

　Section 2　　Hospice Care ·· 107

　　20.2.1　Concept of hospice care ·· 107

　　20.2.2　Development of hospice care ·· 108

　　20.2.3　Research object of hospice care ·· 108

　　20.2.4　Organizational form and concept of dying patients ···················· 108

　Section 3　　Nursing of Dying Patients ·· 109

　　20.3.1　Physiological changes ··· 109

　　20.3.2　Nursing measures ··· 109

Chapter 21　Stress Management ·· 111

　Section 1　　Overview of Stress and Stressful Events ·· 111

　　21.1.1　Overview of stress ··· 111

　　21.1.2　Common stressful events ··· 112

　Section 2　　Response and Harm of Stress ·· 113

　　21.2.1　Stress response ·· 113

　　21.2.2　Harm of stress to the human body ··· 114

　Section 3　　Stress Management of Nurses ·· 115

　　21.3.1　Main source of nurses' stress ··· 115

　　21.3.2　Stress management methods ··· 116

第一章　护理心理学概述 ·· 117

　第一节　护理心理学简介 ·· 117

　　一、心理学的概念 ··· 117

　　二、护理心理学的概念 ·· 117

　　三、护理心理学的意义 ·· 117

　　四、护理心理学的研究任务 ··· 118

　第二节　心理学重要的理论 ·· 119

　　一、心理动力学理论 ·· 119

二、行为主义理论 ………………………………………………………… 119

三、人本主义理论 ………………………………………………………… 120

四、认知理论 ……………………………………………………………… 120

第二章　发展心理学概述 …………………………………………………… 122

第一节　发展心理学研究概述 …………………………………………… 122

一、成长 …………………………………………………………………… 122

二、发展 …………………………………………………………………… 122

三、个体发展阶段 ………………………………………………………… 122

第二节　个体成长和发展的原则及其影响因素 ………………………… 124

一、发展的原则 …………………………………………………………… 124

二、影响个体发展的因素 ………………………………………………… 124

三、影响个体生长发育的因素 …………………………………………… 124

第三章　婴儿的发展 ………………………………………………………… 126

第一节　婴儿的生理发展 ………………………………………………… 126

一、婴儿的身体发展 ……………………………………………………… 126

二、婴儿的动作发展 ……………………………………………………… 127

第二节　婴儿的认知发展 ………………………………………………… 127

一、感知觉发展 …………………………………………………………… 127

二、注意的发生发展 ……………………………………………………… 128

第三节　婴儿情绪、社会性发展 ………………………………………… 128

一、情绪发展 ……………………………………………………………… 128

二、婴儿情绪的社会化 …………………………………………………… 128

第四节　婴儿的护理 ……………………………………………………… 129

第四章　幼儿的发展 ………………………………………………………… 131

第一节　幼儿的生理、认知发展 ………………………………………… 131

一、幼儿的生理发展 ……………………………………………………… 131

二、幼儿的认知发展 ……………………………………………………… 131

第二节　幼儿期情感和人格发展 ………………………………………… 132

一、家长情感陪护 ………………………………………………………… 132

二、依恋行为与分离焦虑 ………………………………………………… 132

三、幼儿的独立意识 ……………………………………………………… 132

第三节　幼儿的健康护理 ………………………………………………… 133

一、身体护理 ……………………………………………………………… 133

二、社会能力护理 ………………………………………………………… 133

三、心理护理 ……………………………………………………………… 133

第五章 　学龄前期儿童的发展 ·· 135

　第一节 　学龄前期儿童的生理发展 ·································· 135

　　一、身体发展 ·· 135

　　二、大脑发育 ·· 135

　　三、运动发展 ·· 135

　第二节 　学龄前期儿童的认知发展 ·································· 136

　　一、语言发展 ·· 136

　　二、注意力发展特点 ·· 136

　　三、想象力发展特点 ·· 136

　　四、思维的发展 ·· 136

　第三节 　学龄前期儿童的心理发展 ·································· 137

　　一、主动对内疚的冲突 ··· 137

　　二、自我意识的发展 ·· 137

　第四节 　学龄前期儿童的情绪发展 ·································· 138

　　一、移情能力迅速发展 ··· 138

　　二、情绪理解依存于社会知识 ······································ 138

　第五节 　学龄前期儿童健康评估和护理 ························· 138

　　一、营养 ··· 138

　　二、日常活动 ·· 139

　　三、保护牙齿 ·· 139

第六章 　学龄期儿童的发展 ··· 140

　第一节 　学龄期儿童的生理发展 ···································· 140

　第二节 　学龄期儿童的心理发展 ···································· 141

　　一、勤奋与自卑的冲突 ··· 141

　　二、学龄期儿童的认知发展 ··· 141

　第三节 　学龄期儿童情绪和性格发展 ····························· 142

　　一、学龄期儿童的情绪发展 ··· 142

　　二、学龄期儿童的性格发展 ··· 142

　第四节 　学龄期儿童身心护理 ······································· 142

　　一、身体护理 ·· 143

　　二、心理护理 ·· 143

第七章 　青少年的发展 ·· 144

　第一节 　青少年的生理发展 ·· 144

　　一、身体外形的变化 ·· 144

　　二、体内生理功能的增强 ·· 145

　　　　三、性的发育和成熟 ································· 145

　　第二节　青少年的心理发展 ························· 146

　　　　一、自我意识的发展 ····························· 146

　　　　二、情绪发展特点 ······························· 147

　　　　三、人际交往特点 ······························· 147

　　第三节　青少年的认知发展 ························· 147

　　第四节　青少年的身心护理 ························· 148

　　　　一、心理护理 ··································· 148

　　　　二、身体护理 ··································· 148

第八章　成年早中期个体的发展 ····················· 150

　　第一节　成年早期个体的概述 ······················· 150

　　　　一、成年早期的年龄规定 ························· 150

　　　　二、成年早期的一般特征 ························· 150

　　　　三、成年早期的认知特点 ························· 150

　　第二节　成年中期个体的概述 ······················· 151

　　第三节　成年早中期个体护理和健康计划 ············· 152

　　　　一、心理护理 ··································· 152

　　　　二、身体护理 ··································· 152

第九章　成年晚期个体的发展 ······················· 154

　　第一节　成年晚期的认知特点 ······················· 154

　　　　一、感知觉发生显著的退行性变化 ················· 154

　　　　二、记忆随增龄而减退 ··························· 155

　　　　三、思维的变化 ································· 155

　　第二节　成年晚期的情绪情感特点 ··················· 155

　　　　一、比较容易产生消极的情绪情感 ················· 155

　　　　二、情感体验深刻而持久 ························· 155

　　第三节　成年晚期的护理工作 ······················· 156

　　　　一、成年晚期常见健康问题 ······················· 156

　　　　二、成年晚期护理保健措施 ······················· 156

第十章　学习 ··································· 158

　　第一节　学习的概念 ····························· 158

　　　　一、学习过程 ··································· 158

　　　　二、新生儿的学习 ······························· 158

　　第二节　早期学习理论 ··························· 159

　　　　一、经典条件反射 ······························· 159

　　二、操作性条件反射 ··· 160

　　三、社会学习理论 ··· 163

第十一章　智力 ··· 165

　第一节　智力的概述 ··· 165

　　一、智力理论 ··· 165

　　二、多元智能理论 ··· 165

　第二节　智力和智商 ··· 166

　第三节　情商 ··· 167

第十二章　动机 ··· 169

　第一节　动机的概述 ··· 169

　　一、动机行为 ··· 169

　　二、动机模型 ··· 169

　第二节　动机的分类与相关理论 ··· 170

　　一、动机的分类 ··· 170

　　二、人本主义理论 ··· 171

　第三节　临床护理中的应用 ··· 172

　　一、需要在临床护理中的应用 ·· 172

　　二、动机在临床护理中的应用 ·· 172

第十三章　情绪 ··· 174

　第一节　情绪的概念及要素 ··· 174

　　一、情绪的概念 ··· 174

　　二、情绪的要素 ··· 174

　第二节　情绪的发展及影响因素 ··· 175

　　一、情绪的发展 ··· 175

　　二、影响情绪发展的因素 ·· 175

第十四章　记忆 ··· 177

　第一节　记忆的概念与分类 ··· 177

　　一、记忆的概念 ··· 177

　　二、记忆的分类 ··· 178

　第二节　遗忘 ··· 179

　　一、遗忘的进程 ··· 179

　　二、遗忘的原因 ··· 179

第十五章　人格 ··· 181

　第一节　人格的定义及研究意义 ··· 181

　　一、人格的定义 ··· 181

二、研究人格的意义 ………………………………………………… 181

第二节　人格的发展 …………………………………………………… 182

一、行为主义者认为人格特质的 3 个方面 ……………………… 182

二、精神分析方法 ………………………………………………… 182

三、人本主义的理论 ……………………………………………… 184

第十六章　疾病 ………………………………………………………… 186

第一节　概述 …………………………………………………………… 186

一、基本概念 ……………………………………………………… 186

二、疾病的分类 …………………………………………………… 187

三、影响疾病的因素 ……………………………………………… 187

四、疾病阶段 ……………………………………………………… 187

五、疾病对患者、家庭和社会的影响 …………………………… 188

第二节　患者角色与护士承担的角色 ………………………………… 189

一、患者角色 ……………………………………………………… 189

二、恶性肿瘤患者的心理反应 …………………………………… 190

三、护士承担的角色 ……………………………………………… 190

第十七章　残疾 ………………………………………………………… 192

第一节　概述 …………………………………………………………… 192

一、残疾的概念 …………………………………………………… 192

二、护理人员学习残疾的意义 …………………………………… 192

三、残疾分类 ……………………………………………………… 192

四、导致残疾的主要原因 ………………………………………… 193

第二节　残疾的心理反应阶段 ………………………………………… 193

第十八章　住院治疗 …………………………………………………… 195

第一节　概述 …………………………………………………………… 195

一、住院的定义 …………………………………………………… 195

二、心理护理的程序 ……………………………………………… 195

第二节　不同年龄阶段住院患者的心理特点 ………………………… 196

一、儿童患者的心理特点 ………………………………………… 196

二、青年患者的心理特点 ………………………………………… 196

三、中年患者的心理特点 ………………………………………… 196

四、老年患者的心理特点 ………………………………………… 197

第三节　情绪问题的心理护理 ………………………………………… 197

一、焦虑 …………………………………………………………… 197

二、抑郁 …………………………………………………………… 198

三、恐惧 ·· 198

四、愤怒 ·· 198

第十九章　损失和哀伤 ·· 201

　第一节　损失 ·· 201

　　一、损失的定义 ·· 201

　　二、损失的类型 ·· 202

　第二节　哀伤 ·· 202

　　一、哀伤的定义 ·· 202

　　二、哀伤的类型 ·· 203

　　三、哀伤的阶段 ·· 203

　　四、帮助哀伤的人 ·· 204

　第三节　在医疗环境中的损失和悲伤 ·· 204

　　一、与临终的成年患者交流 ·· 204

　　二、与临终的患儿交流 ·· 205

　　三、急诊科中的死亡 ·· 205

第二十章　临终护理 ·· 207

　第一节　濒死和死亡 ·· 207

　　一、概念 ·· 207

　　二、死亡标准 ·· 207

　　三、死亡过程的分期 ·· 207

　第二节　临终关怀 ·· 208

　　一、概念 ·· 208

　　二、临终关怀的发展 ·· 208

　　三、临终关怀的研究对象 ·· 208

　　四、临终关怀的组织形式和理念 ·· 208

　第三节　临终患者的生理变化及护理 ·· 209

　　一、生理变化 ·· 209

　　二、护理措施 ·· 209

第二十一章　压力管理 ·· 212

　第一节　压力的概述及压力事件 ·· 212

　　一、压力的概述 ·· 212

　　二、常见的压力事件 ·· 213

　第二节　压力的反应及损害 ·· 213

　　一、压力的反应 ·· 213

　　二、压力对人体的危害 ·· 214

第三节　护士的压力管理 ……………………………………………………… 215

　　一、护士压力的主要来源 ……………………………………………… 215

　　二、压力管理的方法 …………………………………………………… 215

参考文献 ………………………………………………………………… 217

第三节　护士的压力管理

　　一、护士压力的主要来源

　　二、压力管理的方法

Chapter 1 Overview of Nursing Psychology

Summary

Objectives

1. Master the concepts of psychology and nursing psychology.
2. Get familiar with research tasks in nursing psychology.
3. Understand the relevant theories of psychology.

Section 1 Introduction to Nursing Psychology

1.1.1 Concept of psychology

Psychology comes from the Greek word "psyche", meaning "heart" and "mind"; "logos", meaning "knowledge" and "ideas". Psychology is the study of human behavior, thought processes, and emotions. Behavior is the way an organism adapts to its environment. Divided into two categories, explicit behavior and implicit behavior. Explicit behavior refers to directly observable behaviors and responses. Such as eating, talking. Implicit behavior refers to internal activities. For example, thinking, dreaming, and memory. Mental processes, or cognitive processes, refer to all the ways in which we understand the world around us. Emotional process refers to people's attitude experience and corresponding behavioral response to objective things.

Psychologists conduct basic research to describe, explain, predict, and control behavior. Applied psychologists have a purpose—to improve the quality of human life.

1.1.2 Concept of nursing psychology

Nursing psychology is an applied discipline that studies how to use psychological theories, techniques and methods to solve psychological problems in nursing practice in order to achieve the best nursing. It is an interdisciplinary subject formed by the combination of psychology and nursing.

1.1.3 Significance of nursing psychology

1.1.3.1 Comprehensively improve the quality of care

The object of nursing is people, people have complex psychological activities, and it is necessary to understand people's psychological activities in order to satisfy the service object. Nurses have learned nursing psychology, mastered the laws of patients' psychological activities, and fully understood the diseases and patients. Only then can they adopt corresponding psychological nursing techniques for psychological nursing, and such nursing will make patients feel physically comfortable and psychologically. This good psychological state of the patient can promote its good physiological function, which in turn promotes the formation of a good and positive psychological state. This positive interaction of physiology and psychology promotes the development of the disease course to a healthy direction, thereby comprehensively and effectively improving the quality of care.

1.1.3.2 Cultivate the good psychological quality of nurses

The new nursing environment requires nurses to have good psychological quality, quick thinking, rich imagination, precise language skills, moderate emotional appeal and good communication skills. However, nurses are also ordinary people, each with their own temperament and personality characteristics. They are also affected by their own physical, psychological, and social changes. Various emotional and psychological changes may occur. For example, if the psychological state is not well adjusted, to a certain extent negative impact on nursing work and its quality. Therefore, nurses should consciously adjust their psychological state and re-cultivate and optimize their professional psychological quality. Under the theoretical guidance of nursing psychology, they should continuously strengthen professional learning and practice in practice, and strive to make themselves skilled in professional skills, perfect in knowledge structure and professional in practice. Nursing workers with excellent psychological quality.

1.1.4 Research tasks of nursing psychology

As an independent discipline that has just emerged, nursing psychology has an incomplete theoretical system framework. In order to meet the needs of modern social development, efforts must be made to improve the theoretical system and constantly explore scientific application models to guide nursing practice and clinical work. The research tasks of nursing psychology are particularly important, including the following tasks.

1.1.4.1 To study the laws and characteristics of the psychological changes of nursing objects in nursing practice

Individuals' congenital heredity and acquired environment are different, and the personality psychology formed is different. Therefore, there are great differences in the psychological reactions of nursing objects in nursing practice. Generally speaking, no matter what disease a patient has, it will have a certain negative impact on the patient's psychological activities, especially if they suffer from some acute, serious, difficult to cure and poor prognosis diseases. However, different nursing objects have different psychological changes and psychological reactions due to differences in personality and psychology. For example, when they know they have cancer, introverted people often show acute psychological reactions dominated by depression; extroverted people show acute psychological reactions dominated by anger. Therefore, studying the personality psychology of nursing objects is beneficial to improve the effect of psychological nursing.

1.1.4.2 To study the psychological changes of nursing staff in nursing practice

Nursing practice is an interactive process between nursing staff and nursing objects. Nursing staff with noble professional ethics is the premise of psychological nursing, good psychological quality is the basis of psychological nursing, sound personality psychology is the guarantee of psychological nursing, and skilled nursing technology is the condition of psychological nursing. Therefore, the personality and psychological characteristics of nursing staff and the psychological changes in nursing practice will affect the effectiveness of psychological nursing.

1.1.4.3　Research methods of psychological nursing

Nursing is a systematic nursing based on nursing procedures for psychological problems, which is divided into five steps: psychosocial assessment, psychological problem diagnosis, psychological nursing planning, psychological nursing implementation and psychological nursing evaluation. In order to better carry out psychological care in accordance with the nursing procedures, one should be proficient in observation techniques, communication techniques, counseling techniques, psychological assessment and intervention techniques on the basis of a good nurse–patient relationship. Sharp observation can more accurately detect the psychological problems of the nursing object; proper communication can not only understand the nursing object more and faster, but also harmonious the relationship between nursing and patient; sincere consultation can help to change the cognition of nursing object that is not conducive to nursing. The model is also conducive to stimulating their confidence in overcoming the disease; accurate psychological assessment can not only qualitatively and quantitatively assess psychological problems to provide the basis for psychological nursing diagnosis, but also provide objective data for nursing research; exquisite intervention technology helps psychological problems solution or mitigation.

1.1.4.4　Research and apply the content and methods of mental health education

Because mental health is more easily affected by the surrounding environment and the crowd than physical health, and the psychological impact of the patient's physical and psychological status and changes on his relatives is often much greater than the physiological impact, appropriate psychological measures should be taken for patients and their families. Health education is very necessary. Appropriate mental health education for normal people can help people prevent the occurrence of certain psychological problems, or respond in time when psychological problems occur. Appropriate mental health education can also help people to have a correct understanding of certain diseases and eliminate psychological fears caused by misunderstandings.

Section 2　Important Theories of Psychology

Psychologists have many different ways of trying to understand the human mind, and different psychologists have different theories of human behavior from different viewpoints. These views have changed over the years, but the most common are psychodynamic theory, behaviorism theory, humanistic theory, and cognitive theory.

1.2.1　Psychodynamic theory

Psychodynamic theory, also known as psychoanalytic theory, was proposed by Sigmund Freud (1856—1936) at the end of the 19th century, and then developed by Erickson, Jung, and Klein. A key component of psychodynamics is the internal or unconscious conflict that motivates one's behavior. It is believed that childhood experiences are crucial to the formation of adult personality. Freud divided the human psychological structure into three levels: consciousness, subconsciousness and preconsciousness, and vividly compared it to an iceberg floating on the sea.

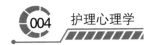

1.2.1.1 Consciousness

It refers to the mental part that an individual can perceive in a state of awakening, which can be perceived by self-consciousness, and it is only a limited external part of individual mental activity. Consciousness can maintain an individual's perception of the environment and self-state, and plays an important role in human adaptation. Freud once made an analogy, thinking that the conscious part of mental activity is like the tip of an iceberg above sea level, while the subconscious is the huge part of the iceberg that can not be seen below the ocean.

1.2.1.2 Subconsciousness

Also known as the unconsciousness, it refers to the part of the mind that the individual can not directly perceive when he is awake, such as unpleasant childhood experiences that have been forgotten by consciousness, psychological trauma, unsatisfied emotional experiences and instincts, desires and Impulsivity, the subconscious content is generally not acceptable to external reality, morality, reason, etc.

1.2.1.3 Preconsciousness

Between the conscious and the subconscious, it refers to the part of the mind that is not currently conscious, but can be brought to the conscious level through focused attention or reminders. The role of the preconscious is to control desires and needs, so that they can be adjusted as much as possible in accordance with the requirements of external reality norms and personal morality. It is a buffer zone between consciousness and subconsciousness.

Psychoanalytic theory is the earliest psychological system to systematically explain human psychology and behavior. It has made important contributions to understanding and explaining human psychology and its laws. It is also an important orientation of psychotherapy and is important for maintaining mental health and preventing mental diseases.

1.2.2 Behaviorism theory

Behaviorism theory, also known as "stimulus-response-result" theory, was established by American psychologist John Watson in the 1920s on the basis of Russian psychologist Pavlov's classical conditioning theory of American psychologists Skinner (Frederic Skinner) and Bandura (Albert Bandura) further improved and developed the behaviorist theory.

Beginning at the end of the 19th century, the Russian physiologist Pavlov conducted a famous experimental study of conditioning. The first step of the experiment: stimulate the dog's oral cavity to produce salivation response with food. Food is an unconditioned stimulus, and the reflex process of saliva secretion is called unconditioned reflex. Unconditioned reflex is an instinctive behavior, not self-learning. For example, babies have sucking reflexes and hugging reflexes after birth. The second step of the experiment: every time the dog was given food, it was always accompanied by a bell, that is, the food was always paired with another neutral environmental stimulus that was not originally related to salivation, such as a bell. The third step of the experiment: after a certain period of training, the bell alone stimulated the salivation of dogs without food. At this point, this neutral stimulus (the bell) becomes a conditioned stimulus. The reflex process of saliva secretion caused by the bell is called conditioned reflex. Behaviors acquired through conditioning can not be manipulated and controlled by individuals at will, and belong to reactive behaviors, also known as classical conditioning.

Operant conditioning theory emphasizes the effect of behavioral outcome C (consequence) on behavior itself. This theory was established by American psychologist Skinner and others through animal experiments. Experiments were carried out in the famous Skinner box. Hungry mice will show a series of blind behaviors in the experimental box, such as screaming, biting, scurrying, pressing the lever. Only after pressing the lever, the mouse can get food, that is, "appearance of food" versus "pressing". The "bar" action has the effect of promoting and strengthening. After many experiments, the rats learned the behavior of pressing the lever to get food, that is, the conditioned reflex was established between operating the lever and getting food. The reinforcing effect of the result (appearance of food) accompanying the behavior (manipulating the lever) on the behavior itself is called reinforcement, and the stimulus result is called the reinforcer. Similarly, in the avoidance manipulation condition experiment, animals receiving electric shocks will produce a series of behavioral responses (such as screaming, biting, scurrying, avoiding), one of which is the avoidance action, which can be withdrawn the result of the electric shock. The result of withdrawing the shock had a reinforcing effect on avoidance behavior, and as a result the animals learned the avoidance behavior. The above experiments show that when a certain behavior (such as pressing a lever or avoiding behavior) occurs, a positive result (appearance of food or withdrawal of electric shock) can always be obtained, and the individual gradually learns to operate on this behavior, which is the operating condition reflection.

Social observation learning theory is Bandura, which emphasizes that people's social behavior is obtained through observational learning, and does not receive direct reinforcement and rewards. Individuals can achieve imitation learning only by observing other people's behavioral responses. In nursing work, the theory has important application value. For example, the formation of the patient's role behavior has a certain relationship with the demonstration role, including shouting, groaning, and coping methods; similarly, the principle of demonstration role can also be used in the guidance and care of patients, as well as in the education of children and patients.

1.2.3   Humanistic theory

Humanistic theory in the 20th century in the United States in the 1950s and 1960s, is represented by Maslow (Abrabo Maslow) and Rogers (Karl Rogers), which emphasizes human dignity, value, creativity and self-realization, emphasizing that human beings have potential. The body, self-realization boils down to the development of potential, known as the third force of psychology.

The contribution of humanistic theory is to emphasize the important role of the individual in psychological development, to let the individual realize his own nature, to determine his own behavior by his own will, to repair the damaged self-realization potential, and to promote the healthy development of the individual. The client-centered therapy developed on this basis is also one of the leading therapies in the current psychological counseling and therapy.

1.2.4   Cognitive theory

Cognitive theory originated in the 1950s and is closely related to the development of cognitive psychology. Cognitive psychology mainly studies the information processing process of human cognition, and uses it to explain complex human behaviors, such as concept formation, problem solving, language and emotion. Cognitive theory holds that cognition plays a decisive role in emotion and behavior, and that thoughts and beliefs are the causes of emotional states and behavioral manifestations. On this basis, American psychologists Ellis (Albert Ellis) and Baker (A. T. Beck) put forward the ABC theory of emotion and the cognitive theory of emotional disorders respectively, and developed the corresponding theory and technology of cognitive therapy.

Chapter 2 Overview of Developmental Psychology

> **Objectives**
> 1. Master the factors that influence growth and development.
> 2. Become familiar with the field of human development and the principles of development.
> 3. Understand the concept of human growth and development.

Section 1　Overview of Developmental Psychology Research

2.1.1　Growth

Growth generally refers to growing up and becoming an adult, and also generally refers to the process of things becoming mature and getting rid of immaturity. To put it simply, it is a process of change in which oneself continues to become mature and stable. Growth is approaching in a direction that is the age of a particular powerful person in the social circle in which the individual is located. Generally speaking, our interpretation of growth is the experience of an individual's physical and psychological development towards maturity.

Among the three conditions, physical maturity is the material basis for psychological maturity, and social maturity is a necessary condition for psychological maturity. The improvement of the degree of socialization depends on the social practice activities of individuals.

2.1.2　Development

Change process of things from small to large, from simple to complex, from low-level to high-level, and from old material to new material. Psychology believes that human development refers to the changing process of all laws in the body and mind from birth to death, and it is a process from multi-level quantitative change to qualitative change. It includes two aspects: physiological development and psychological development. ①Physhological development: refers to the development of various tissue systems (bones, muscles, heart, nervous system, respiratory system, etc.). ②Psychological development: refers to the regular psychological changes of individuals, including the development of knowledge, intelligence and intention.

2.1.3　Stage of individual development

The first stage: conception to birth. This stage, also known as the prenatal period, develops from a

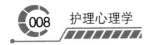

fertilized egg to an embryo, to a fetus, and finally to the birth of a newborn.

The second stage: birth to one year old. This stage is also known as the infancy or neonatal period. Considered the most important of all, and the one that can not be ignored, this stage focuses on the development of a good attachment relationship between the child and the mother and other primary caregivers. Parents' ways of raising their children and their attitudes towards children should be based on a regular basis. The way of feeding, caring and attitude towards children should not be such that children often experience an uncertainty. At the same time this period, the baby-like self, is optimistic and confident about life, brave, and has a strong desire to explore the world and self-realization.

The third stage: 1-6 years old. This period is the childhood of the child. Mainly to solve children's autonomy, independent development, and compliance with life rules, social norms. During this period, the child's cognitive ability begins to develop, the child's self-awareness begins to form, the child is in the first resistance period, the development of autonomy and independence is very important for the child's life, but the child must also learn to obey living norms and social rules, which are often many parents tossing about these two issues, whether it is looser or stricter, parents often do not know how to deal with it. At this stage, the child's imagination and creativity are mainly developed.

The fourth stage: 6-12 years old, also known as childhood. This stage is mainly to form a child's sense of diligence and responsibility. We know that these two qualities are very important for life. If a child possesses both qualities, parents need not worry about their child's life. We say that the children of the poor are in charge of their homes early. These children learn from an early age that they are responsible for themselves and others. Very diligent to study and work. They have enough self-sufficiency and self-protection ability and wisdom, and gradually get rid of the interference and influence of their parents and society, and seek self-independence and openness. Dare to be authentic, innate, and pure. At this time, the client will become more and more confident, brave and responsible, as well as relaxed and happy.

The fifth stage: around 13 years old to adulthood, which is what we call adolescence. Erickson thinks it is the stage of character identification, the stage of identity. It is the final stage of the child's journey to adulthood, and the stage in which all preparations for adulthood are made. It is also the most confusing and headache stage in the industrialized society in the world. Psychological problems often arise because the client is stuck in childhood. I still feel that I am weak and do not have the ability and wisdom to be self-sufficient and self-protective. Continue to use the old strategy for sustenance and protection. What is shown are low self-esteem, do not believe in yourself; timid, lack of courage; shirk, dare not take responsibility. Specific psychological problems are anxiety, fear, compulsion, depression and contradictions, conflicts.

Therefore, we must use active attention, serious listening, deep understanding, and unconditional acceptance to create a safe, warm, and relaxed atmosphere for children, so that children can be their true self, fully express themselves, and be seen and heard. Respect, understand, accept, recognize, support and appreciate, gradually become yourself, and gain the confidence and courage to be yourself. Then, together with the children, gradually discover and develop their own abilities and wisdom, and develop more adult, more effective strategies for feeding and protecting themselves. Encourage children to gradually become an optimistic, confident, courageous, daring, active, active, capable and wise person. The most direct effect of this is that the person concerned is no longer so anxious, fearful, depressed or self-compulsive, as well as a happy personal and family life, career success and interpersonal harmony.

The sixth stage: adulthood is the age group of 25-60 years old. According to the psychological and physiological characteristics of adults, it can be divided into three stages: late adolescence (25 – 30 years old), early adulthood (30 – 40 years old), and middle adulthood (40 – 60 years old). In adulthood, the human body matures and various physiological activities are relatively stable. As far as the development of the brain is concerned, the maturation process of the brain has been basically completed before the age of 20, but some aspects are still developing. The process of myelination is an important indicator of brain development, and the process of myelination of the reticular tissue continues into the 30s. The brain association area, which is the physiological basis of intellectual processes, develops into old age. But with age, the functions of various organ systems in the human body begin to decline. Especially after middle adulthood, various functions of the body, such as physical strength, energy, and disease resistance, show a downward trend and become more and more obvious with age. Therefore, late youth and early adulthood are the golden period of life, with strong physical strength and energy, rich social experience and cultural knowledge, and become the basic force of various social undertakings, production and activities, and the main bearer of family care for the elderly. Cherish this time.

The final stage: aging. Biologically speaking, aging is a spontaneous and inevitable process of organisms with the passage of time. It is a complex natural phenomenon, which is manifested as structural degeneration, functional decline, and reduced adaptability and resistance. Physiologically, aging is viewed as an ontogeny from the fertilized egg to old age. Pathologically, aging is the result of the accumulation of stress and strain, injury and infection, a decline in immuneresponses, malnutrition, metabolic disorders, and neglect and drug abuse. In addition, from a sociological point of view, aging is a personal loss of interest in new things, detachment from reality, and a fondness for nostalgia. Aging has no clear boundaries and is unavoidable, mainly based on physiological and psychological changes.

Section 2   Principle Factors and Influencing Factors of Individual Growth and Development

2.2.1   Principle of development

Children follow certain rules as they grow and develop.

The principle of head first. Refers to the sequence of development from top tobottom. The development of the child's body strictly follows the sequence of head and neck, trunk, lower limbs. Develop head and upper body abilities first, then develop the rest of the body.

From near to far principle. Refers to the development sequence of the mid – axial to the periphery. The development sequence of children's movements is from the trunk to the limbs, then to the hands and feet, and finally to the small muscle movements of the fingers and toes. Near means near the heart. First develop the trunk and then develop the limbs. Children learn to use the various parts of their bodies, and they follow this principle. For example, learn to swing your arms first, and then learn to use your fingers.

From simple to complex principle. First develop simple skills independently, and then integrate various simple skills to form more complex skills. For example, learn to grasp a spoon first, and then learn to use a spoon to put it in your mouth. The latter, in addition to simple grasping hand skills, also require hand – eye coordination.

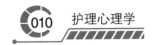

The principle of system independence. Different systems of the human body develop independently at different rates of development. For example, skeletal muscles, nervous system, and sexual organs all belong to different systems with different developmental patterns.

2.2.2 Factors that affect individual development

2.2.2.1 Genetic influence

Inheritance is a physiological phenomenon that refers to the phenomenon in which various characteristics of the body structure and function of the parents are passed on to the next generation through genetics. Inherited biological characteristics, or hereditary qualities, mainly refer to the anatomical and physiological characteristics of the innate organism's structure, shape, sensory and nervous system. Physiological maturity refers to the degree or level of growth and development of an organism, also known as physiological development.

2.2.2.2 Environmental impact

The environment makes possible the possibility of psychological development provided by heredity, and although heredity provides the possibility of psychological development, this possibility can not become a reality without living in a social environment. Although the children raised by beasts have the genetic qualities of humans, they do not possess the normal psychology of humans. The environment refers to the external world that surrounds the individual and spontaneously influences the individual. That is, the natural and social environment surrounding the individual. This does not include educational activities that intentionally and consciously influence people. It mainly refers to the geographical environment, cultural traditions, customs, political background, social relations and social atmosphere of the family. These all affect a person's development.

2.2.3 Factors affecting individual growth and development

2.2.3.1 Nutrition

Reasonable nutrition is the material basis for children's growth and development, and the younger the age, the greater the impact of nutrition. Intrauterine malnutrition fetuses not only have backward physical growth, but also slow brain development; long-term malnutrition after birth will first lead to no weight gain, and eventually will affect the growth of height and the body's immune, endocrine, neuromodulation and other functions are low, affects the development of intellectual, psychological and social adaptation. Obesity caused by excessive calorie intake in children can also have a serious impact on their growth and development.

2.2.3.2 Diseases and drugs

The impact of disease on the growth and development of children is very obvious. Acute infection often leads to weight loss; long-term chronic diseases affect both weight and height growth; endocrine diseases often cause delayed bone growth and nervous system development; congenital diseases such as congenital heart disease, trisomy 21 syndrome, and neuropsychological development. Some drugs can also affect the growth and development of children, such as streptomycin and gentamicin in larger doses or for a long time, which can cause hearing loss or even deafness; long-term use of adrenal glucocorticoids can slow down the growth rate of height.

2.2.3.3   Pregnant mother situation

The development of the fetus in the womb is affected by factors such as the living environment, nutrition, mood, and health status of the pregnant mother. Such as rubella, herpes zoster, cytomegalovirus infection in early pregnancy, can lead to fetal congenital malformations; severe malnutrition in pregnant mothers can cause miscarriage, premature birth and fetal growth and brain development delay; pregnant mothers receive drugs, radiation environmental pollution and mental trauma, can hinder fetal development. Intrauterine growth arrest can affect the growth and development of children after birth. In addition, pregnant women can convert what she thinks and hears, and even the feelings in dreams, into information about changes in the environment in the fetus, and transmit it to the fetus unknowingly. The nutrients needed for fetal growth and development are provided by the maternal blood circulation through the placenta. The adverse emotional changes of pregnant women will affect the intake of nutrients, the secretion of hormones and the biochemical composition of blood, so that substances in the blood that are harmful to other tissues and organs of the nervous system surge, and affect fetal development through the placenta, thereby causing fetal malformations.

Chapter 3   Development of Infants

Summary

Objectives

1. Learn how to care for babies in the ward or in the community.
2. Physiological and psychological development process of infancy.
3. Master the abnormal reaction of the baby and how to care for it.

Section 1   Physiological Development of Infants

Physiological development of an infant refers to the growth and development of its brain and body in terms of shape, structure and function. The activity of the brain, nervous system and senses is the basis of mental activity. The physiological development of infants directly affects and restricts the occurrence and development of infant physiology, so the development of infant physiology has always been the main subject of research.

3.1.1   Body development of infants

3.1.1.1   Morphological development of the infant brain

(1) Brain weight and head circumference

The baby's brain begins to develop from the embryonic period and weighs 350–400 g at birth, which is 25% of the adult brain weight. After that, the brain weight increased the fastest in the first year, reaching 700–800 g in 6 months and 800–900 g in 12 months. To a certain extent, these developmental changes reflect the development and maturation of the internal structure of the brain at various stages, and are closely related to the development of the cerebral cortex area. At the same time, there are similar developmental changes in infant head circumference. At birth, the head circumference has reached about 34 cm, and at 12 months, it has reached 46–47 cm.

(2) Cerebral cortex

The basic structure of the brain is already in place when the fetus is 6 or 7 months old. At birth, brain cells have been differentiated, cellular structure and hierarchical differentiation have been basically completed, most sulci and gyri have appeared, the insula has been covered by adjacent lobes, and the basic sensorimotor pathways in the brain have been myelinated (except white matter). Since then, infant cortical cells have developed rapidly, expanded hierarchically, decreased neuronal density and differentiated from each other, and increasingly complex synaptic apparatus.

3.1.1.2   Functional development of the infant brain

(1) Electroencephalogram

Changes in Electroencephalogram (EEG) are often used as an important indicator of infant brain development. Studies have confirmed that 5-month-old fetuses have shown EEG activity, and after 8 months, they have the same EEG as newborns. EEG activity begins to have continuity and initial rhythm, forming a brain that sleeps and wakes up electrogram. 5 months after birth is an important stage in the development of infant brain electrical activity. Gradual corticalization of EEG with subcortical inhibition. 5-12 months, the evoked potentials caused by external stimuli change, such as the configuration of visual evoked potentials becomes complicated, and the latency is shortened.

(2) Cortical center

The infant brain develops according to the sequence of its genetic structure, following the head-to-tail principle and the distance principle. When the baby is just born, the two hemispheres of the brain and its cortex can not function normally, and the cortical excitation is still in a diffuse state, so as long as any part of the newborn's body is touched, it will cause the head, hands and feet to move.

3.1.1.3   Process of infant body development and its normal values

The physiological development process of infants refers to the growth and development of structures and functions of various parts of the body and various organs and tissues. Growth refers to the increase in quantity, such as body length, weight and the growth of various organs; development refers to qualitative changes, such as the continuous differentiation and maturation of various organs, tissue structures and functions.

(1) Weight

At birth, a full-term baby boy weighs 3.3-3.4 kg, and a full-term baby girl weighs 3.2-3.3 kg. Under normal feeding, infants doubled their weight by 5 months and tripled by 12 months.

(2) Height

At birth, full-term newborns are about 50 cm tall. Among them, the baby boy is slightly taller than the baby girl, and the first baby is slightly shorter than the second and third baby. At the same time, affected by the size and nutrition of the baby at birth, the growth rate is about 2.54 cm per month in the first year.

(3) Head and tail

When a baby is just born, the head circumference has reached about 34 cm, and at 0-3 months, it will grow by 2 cm per month; at 4-6 months, it will increase by 1 cm per month; at 6-12 months, it will increase by 0.5 cm per month; 1-2 years old, growth of 2 cm a year.

(4) Teeth

Babies' teeth, according to their position, shape and function, can be divided into incisors, canines and deciduous molars. Baby teeth begin to grow at 6-9 months after birth.

3.1.2   Motor development of infants

The development of various movements and movements of infants is the direct premise of the development of their activities, and it is also the external manifestation of their psychological development. The development of infant movements has strict and meticulous internal laws, and follows certain principles. It is a complex and dynamic development system that can be followed regularly.

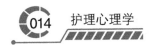

It is generally believed that infant movements first occur in the neonatal period, and their initial unconditioned reflex behavior is the first group of movements that are "first produced". Early human reflex: an organized natural response that occurs automatically when certain stimuli are presented without learning. Sucking and swallowing reflexes: eating. Orientation: find the nipple, cough, sneeze, wink. Babies' ability to control their own muscles continues to increase, and some reflexes will gradually disappear, which will become the basis for mastering more complex behaviors in the future. This stimulates the areas of the brain responsible for complex behaviors, and helps the development of complex behaviors.

Section 2　Cognitive Development of Infants

3.2.1　Development of perception

In the cognitive ability of infants, perception is the first and fastest developing area, and it has always dominated the cognitive activities of infants.

3.2.1.1　Occurrence of vision

A large number of studies have confirmed that the initial occurrence of vision is in the middle and late stages of the fetus, and the 4 – 5 month fetus has the ability to respond to vision and the corresponding physiological basis. Newborns already have certain visual abilities, acquire basic visual processes, and have primitive color vision. For the development of infant vision, relevant studies have confirmed that the color perception of infants 2 – 4 months old has developed very well. In addition, a large number of studies have confirmed that babies at least 6 months have indeed had obvious stereoscopic vision.

3.2.1.2　Occurrence of hearing

In recent years, more and more psychologists believe that, according to their research, normal healthy babies are born with hearing, and hearing can be said to be innate. The latest results of current infant research show that 5 – 6 months old baby has started to build the auditory system and can hear sounds below 1,000 Hz through the mother's body. For the development of hearing acuity, 1 month old infants can distinguish the difference between 200 Hz and 500 Hz pure tones. Infants of 5 – 8 months perceive a 2% change in audio frequency in the range of 1,000 – 3,000 Hz, and the threshold of difference in the range of 4,000 – 8,000 Hz is the same as the adult level. The development of audio – visual coordination: newborn babies have the most basic audio – visual coordination. The 3 – 6 months old infant's audiovisual coordination has developed to a level that enables him to discriminate whether audiovisual information is consistent.

3.2.1.3　Occurrence and development of taste, smell and touch

Taste can already feel enough taste stimulation when infants are 4 months old. The taste of newborns is well developed and occupies a very important position in its defense reflex mechanism. The sense of taste is most developed in infancy and childhood and gradually declines thereafter. At 7 – 8 months, the olfactory receptors of infants are quite mature and have a preliminary olfactory response ability, which can roughly distinguish several different odors. Newborns have been able to make corresponding typical responses to various odors, such as "liking" good smells. They can also establish food conditioning by smell, and can locate the space by preliminary smell. For touch, infants have initial tactile responses at the

49 day, and can respond to fine and sharp stimuli at 2 months. Newborns can compare nipples with different softness and hardness by oral touch, and at 4 months, they can distinguish nipples of different shapes and degrees of softness at the same time. The instinctive tactile response can be manifested at the time of birth, and after 4 months, the infant has mature reaching behavior, and the visual – touch coordination ability has been developed.

3.2.2   Development of attention

Babies are born with attention. This attention is essentially an innate directional reflex, the initial form of unintentional attention. Newborns have developed selective attention and the ability to scan the outside world.

Infants between 1 and 3 months of age have significantly shifted their attention toward curves, irregular shapes of complex stimuli, and all shapes with high contour density. The average attention time of 3 – 6 months infants is shorter and they prefer more complex and meaningful visual objects. After 6 months of age, the babys sleep time decreases, and attention is no longer limited to visual aspects as before, but is more extensive and complex in the form of sucking, grasping and other daily activities.

Section 3   Infant Emotional and Social Development

3.3.1   Emotional development

From birth, an infant is a social person, surrounded by various social objects and social stimuli, forming and developing people's emotions, social behaviors and relationships.

Initial emotional response. After birth, children have emotional manifestations, such as newborn crying, quiet, and limbs kicking. At the same time, the emotional responses of newborn babies have been initially differentiated. Emotion expert Izzard research shows that human babies display five different emotions at birth, namely surprise, sadness, disgust, smile and interest. Research by Chinese psychologist Meng Zhaolan shows that newborns have four expressions of interest, disgust, pain and smile. It can be seen that the baby not only has emotions after birth, but also has been initially differentiated.

3.3.2   Socialization of infant emotions

The emotions of newborn babies are all physiological, which are a kind of primitive instinctive responses, which are caused by some suitable and inappropriate stimuli inside and outside the body, and reflect the internal state and physiological needs of the collective at that time. Infant social smiling, stranger anxiety, separation anxiety, and emotional social referencing are central to infant emotional socialization.

Section 4   Nursing Care of Babies

As a nurse, building trust with your baby is important. According to Erickson's theory of personality development, infancy is a period of conflict between basic trust and distrust. In infancy, don't think that the baby is an ignorant little animal at this time, as long as it is full and does not cry, this is a big mistake. This is a period of psychological conflict between basic trust and distrust, because during this period, the child begins to know people. When the child is crying or hungry, whether the parents appear is an important issue to build trust. Trust forms the quality of "hope" in the personality, which acts as a self-enhancing power. Children with a sense of trust are hopeful, idealistic, and have a strong future orientation. On the contrary, they dare not hope, and are constantly worried that their needs will not be met. Erickson defines hope as: "The enduring belief in the achievability of one's wishes, the roar of rebellion against the forces of darkness, the birth of life."

Therefore, the care of the baby at this stage includes the following ways.

3.4.1　Satisfy sucking needs

By sucking, the baby not only gets food, but also gets a sense of security. From birth to 1 year old, if parents find that their baby has this need, they can use a pacifier to meetit. After your baby can walk, many novelties in the environment will distract him from the pacifier, so there is no need to worry too much about not being able to wean off the pacifier. Due to the strong demand for exploration, babies under the age of one and a half like to stuff whatever they can get into their mouths, which sometimes makes parents nervous. In fact, when the baby's mouth comes into contact with things of different hardness, size and touch, it can stimulate the development of his sensory ability, so generally do not prohibit the baby from sucking.

3.4.2　Establish eating habits

After the baby begins to grow teeth, it is necessary to train to eat complementary food. The chewing process of complementary food is also to meet the baby's oral needs. At this time, it is necessary to cultivate the baby's good eating habits, including fixed meal times, non-partial eclipse, willingness to try foods with different tastes, and focus on eating. Since chewing is one of the ways for babies to meet their needs during the oral stage, eating complementary foods can help babies transition smoothly to the solid food stage, and it will transfer his needs for nipples, pacifiers and feeding bottles, so there will be no over-reliance on pacifiers.

3.4.3　Don't begrudge your hugs

Many people think that it is not good to hold a baby as soon as it cries, and it is easy to develop a personality that is overly dependent on the baby, but this is not the case. Please don't be stingy to hug your baby. When he really needs hugs, parents' hugs and comforts not only bring warm care to the baby, but also enhance his trust in the world, eliminate the insecurity in his heart, and have a great impact on the development of the child's life.

At the same time, different psychological care should be taken for different infants and young children. Some children are quiet and easy to satisfy. Some need more love and care, so the caregiver should be loving, confident, calm and patient to communicate with the child more, so that it has a sense of security and settles down.

Chapter 4   Development of Young Children

Summary

Objectives
1. Understand the psychological characteristics of young children development.
2. Master the characteristics of physical, cognitive, social and emotional development in early childhood.
3. Master child care work.

Section 1   Physiological and Cognitive Development of Young Children

4.1.1   Physical development of young children

For the characteristics of early childhood growth and development, from one year old to 3 years old is young children. The growth and development rate of infancy is the fastest stage in human life, and the growth and development rate of young children after the age of 1 begins to slow down. But the growth is still fast compared to other periods. After the age of 1, children's intelligence and activity are developing rapidly, mainly manifested in many important changes in the structure of the body, and the children's curiosity continues to grow, gradually develop independent consciousness and continue to explore the environment.

4.1.2   Cognitive development of young children

Children at the age of 1–3 are in the unconditional acceptance period. During this period, children's living environment is mainly family, and the most contact is with parents. The requirements of society for children include basic life skills, sensory motor skills development, use of language skills and communication skills, such as recognizing objects and people, learning to eat, learning to control urine, expressing their own requirements in words, addressing people, and following orders or executions some simple instructions.

4.1.2.1   Development of perceptual ability

Sensory ability and perception ability are two different abilities, but they are closely related. Sensation is a cognitive process that reflects the individual attributes of current objective things, such as the sound, color, cold, heat, softness, hardness of an object. The earliest skin sensations (touch, pain,

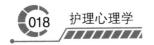

temperature) appear in young children, and then gradually develop a keen sense of smell, taste, vision and hearing.

Perception is a cognitive process that reflects the overall characteristics of current objective things, and it is formed on the basis of perception. Any objective thing contains various attributes, which can not be grasped by a certain feeling alone. When the baby is about 6 months old and can sit up, it can better complete the activities of eye-hand coordination. Under the adjustment of vision, the hand completes the activities of manipulating and fiddling with objects within the field of vision, which is the characteristic of using perceptual ability to comprehensively recognize objects. Until the age of 3, it is a period of rapid development of various perceptual abilities.

4.1.2.2　Improvement of athletic ability

During this period, children learn to walk, begin to speak, and perform activities that are unique to humans such as surface thinking and imagination. Independence emerges. All kinds of psychological activities are gradually complete. The main features are learn to walk upright and use tools. There is a process for children aged 1-3 years to learn practical tools, which generally goes through four stages. In the first stage, the action is not dominated by the characteristics of the tool at all. In the second stage, the new method is no longer continuously changed, and the time for performing the same action is prolonged. In the third stage, take the initiative to repeat effective actions. In the fourth stage, it can be used according to the characteristics of the appliance, and the action mode can be changed according to the objective conditions of use. 2-3 years old can learn a variety of movements, not only the coordination of hands, but also the movement of the whole body and limbs.

4.1.2.3　Strong curiosity

Because of their active nature, strong curiosity, lack of life experience, and poor comprehensive judgment, young children are particularly prone to accidents. Common accidents for infants and young children include falls, accidentally swallowing foreign objects, burns (scalding), electric shocks, gas poisoning, food poisoning and car accidents. For example, some parents do not tell their children clearly in order not to give their children alcohol or touch other liquids. As a result, the children are curious about what good things the parents have hidden, and they secretly drink it without the parents noticing, resulting in food poisoning. Some children are curious to plug chopsticks, toothpicks and other fine objects into the nasal cavity and ear cavity, causing accidents from time to time.

Section 2　Emotional and Personality Development in Early Childhood

4.2.1　Parents' emotional support

The relationship with others is crucial to children's emotional and personality development, and has a strong relationship with children's behavior, satisfaction, self-worth and sense of security. 0-3 years old is a critical period for children to establish emotional dependence. Children at this age are very dependent on their parents. If children change their parents for a long time, it will be difficult for them to trust others.

Children in this period need emotional support from their parents. Children at this age are more sensitive and therefore should not entrust their education to others. For example, when children grow up, they will feel that if they give their parents enough money, they will be happy. This is the same as the love parents have for their children when they are young. Children in the emotional upbringing period must be cultivated by the parents themselves so that the grown-up children can have a rich emotional experience.

4.2.2   Attachment behavior and separation anxiety

Another important aspect of 3-year-old children's personality development is the formation and development of attachment behavior. Attachment behaviors generally refer to the tendency and behavior of infants and young children to seek and maintain close relationships with their caregivers (usually parents). The formation and development of attachment behaviors have a significant impact on future socialization and interpersonal development. Since the formation and development of attachment behaviors are bidirectional, on the one hand, infants and young children seek protection, intimacy and attachment to their parents; on the other hand, parents care and attach to infants and young children. Children understand the world and form personality characteristics such as trust and distrust, security and insecurity. For example, infants and young children raised in isolation (children in orphanages) are limited in the formation and development of attachment behavior due to lack of communication with others. When they grow up, they may appear indifference to others, loneliness, lack of social interaction and other personality characteristics.

4.2.3   Children's sense of independence

American psychologists have tracked 1,500 children for a long time and found that 20% of them had not achieved much after 30 years. Compared with the top 20% of people, the most significant difference is not in intelligence, but in personality qualities. High achievers are people with personality qualities such as perseverance, independence, and courage. It can be seen how important the child's independent character is to growth and maturity.

This stage of personality development is characterized by the initial formation of children's self-concept, knowing the difference between themselves and others, and showing the characteristics of various basic emotional activities, such as anxiety, fear, shyness, hostility and anger. The introverted or extroverted character of the character is also gradually evident at this stage. According to Erickson, children face a crisis of trust and a crisis of autonomy during this period. If the child is properly cared for around the age of 1, such as the satisfaction of the necessary physical and emotional needs from the warmth, care and love of the parents, the child will form a sense of trust, the crisis will be resolved, and the quality of hope will emerge.

Section 3   Health Care for Young Children

Health care for young children includes the following three points: physical, social capability and psychological care. Starting from these aspects is more conducive to children's formation of healthy self-awareness, cultivating their independence, and better preparation for adapting to social life.

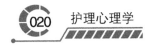

4.3.1 Physical care

Physical care for young children includes weight, height, vital signs, vision and hearing.

Studies have shown that 1 – 3 years old is a critical period for the rapid development of young children's brains. The brain weight of a newborn is about 25% of that of an adult (350–400 g), that of a 1–year–old baby is equivalent to 50% of adults, and that of a 2–year–old baby, the weight of the brain is about 75% of that of an adult, and the brain weight of a 3–year–old baby is close to that of an adult. This shows that after the child is 3 years old, the intelligence quotient, physical fitness, personality and other aspects are almost stereotyped. There are 14 billion nerve cells, also known as "neurons", in the human cerebral cortex. Connections are formed between neurons called "neural circuits". The richer the neural circuits, the more active the brain and the smarter its behavior.

If parents can provide children with rich visual, auditory, tactile, movement and balance stimuli in a timely manner at the age of 1 – 3, the higher the neural circuit density of children's brains, the more intelligent children will be. Without environmental stimulation, the brain development of young children isstunted, the brain weight can be reduced by 20%, and the density of brain neural circuits will also be greatly affected. After the critical period of 1–3 years old, it is difficult for parents to make up for this loss for young children, which means that the brain development of children aged 1 – 3 is an irreversible process.

For a young child to sleep, the brain must be allowed to relax in order to develop and "digest" what it has learned. Therefore, newborns sleep about 20 h a day, and children after 1 year old need to maintain 12–15 h.

4.3.2 Social capability care

For children aged 1–3, parents can appropriately take them to the outdoors to learn about the outside world, and can take them to the garden for a walk. Although children may not be able to speak very well, the stimulation of children by external things can make them better development, so that their development is well promoted. For children aged 3 – 4, parents can take their children to places such as zoos or aquariums, which can not only increase their knowledge but also promote the parent – child relationship between parents and children. You can also take children to learn about public welfare and lead them to understand the spirit of dedication, which not only enriches children's lives, but also lays a good foundation for the construction of children's values.

4.3.3 Psychological care

4.3.3.1 Avoid accusations

Even if a child makes a mistake, there are better ways to educate them than to blame. Try not to use negative words to educate children, it will discourage their initiative.

4.3.3.2 Establishing rules

1–3 years old will always come up with some "disrespectful" words, the parent should not laugh it off because of fun, but tell them seriously, it is wrong to say this, there is no rules and there is no circle, correct them as soon as possible. Otherwise, you will have many rude, annoying little troubles in your life.

4.3.3.3　Restraining behaviors

1−3 years old sometimes make unreasonable demands to adults. Caregivers should treat them carefully and correctly according to their requirements, and let children understand that everyone should restrain their own behavior, not everything can be done.

4.3.3.4　Parents agree on parenting

When parenting children, adults must maintain a consensus, and there must be no red−faced and white−faced role differentiation, and try not to divide opinions.

4.3.3.5　Cultivate the love of children

For the main caregivers of children aged 1 − 3 years, they must have a kind heart and set up role models for them, so that children can imitate and experience the love of their parents, and gradually get love.

4.3.3.6　Cultivating beliefs

Although children can't talk about beliefs, care givers must let them have naive plans and desires to achieve, and are willing to spend time and energy for this. Parents should also satisfy their desires accordingly.

Chapter 5 Development of Preschool Children

Summary

Objectives
1. Master the health assessment and care of preschool children.
2. Understand the cognitive, social and emotional development characteristics of preschool children.
3. Understand the physiological development of preschool children.

Section 1   Physiological Development of Preschool Children

5.1.1   Body development

At this stage, height and weight rise in waves. After the age of 2, the growth rate gradually slows down, with an average annual increase of 4 – 5 cm in height and 5 – 6 kg in weight. Bones, which develop rapidly, have about 45 new epiphysis, the growth points where cartilage becomes epiphysis. The reproductive system begins to slow down at the age of 4 and develops rapidly until adolescence. Circulatory system, lymph glands grow very fast and decline in adolescence (lymph glands help fight infection, promote nutrient absorption, and are good for child health and survival). Digestive system, 20 deciduous teeth appear at the age of 2 and a half, and in late childhood, the deciduous teeth begin to fall out, the stomach capacity is small, and the nutrient intake is rich and high-quality.

5.1.2   Brain development

At this time, in terms of brain development, the weight of the brain reaches 90%, the prefrontal lobe develops rapidly, the function of the cerebellum is gradually strengthened, high-level neural activity, and the autonomic nerve is not fully developed. Rapid development of the prefrontal lobe. The function of the cerebellum is gradually strengthened, which can accurately coordinate various movements and maintain the balance of the body. At the age of 3, the coordination of muscle activity is obviously enhanced; at the age of 5–6, various movements can be performed accurately and coordinated. Advanced neural activity— excited is dominant, the inhibitory process is not perfect, and the exciting process is stronger than the inhibitory process. Hyperactive, easily excited, fatigued, inattentive, easily transferred by external stimuli; the excitation process is strengthened, and the sleep time gradually decreases; strengthen the inhibition process, learn to control their own behavior and carry out various activities more accurately. The autonomic nerves are not fully developed, the sympathetic nerves are highly excitable and the parasympathetic nerves are weaker. For example, the heart rate and respiratory rate are fast, but the rhythm is unstable. Therefore, children's gastrointestinal digestive ability is easily affected by emotions.

5.1.3　Sports development

Preschool children's physical development is rapid, and their athletic ability is greatly improved. Able to keep the body steady and jump forward with both feet continuously. Can hang on the horizontal bar for about 10 s. Can run 15 m with ease. Able to throw sandbags forward about 2 m with one-handed throwing action. Bends the upper body when hopping and hopping on one foot. Able to throw the ball upwards with both hands. Able to walk independently for about 1 km (with appropriate rest on the way). Able to jump forward about 2 m continuously on one foot. Both left and right feet can jump on one foot, and you can alternately go up and down stairs with both feet. He can eat, brush his teeth, wash his face, and learn to wear pullovers, buttons, and zippers by himself. Can practice racket, reach out to catch the ball, throw and kick the ball at the target.

Section 2　Cognitive Development of Preschool Children

5.2.1　Development of language

The research results of children's psychology and long-term educational practice have proved that early childhood is the most rapid and crucial period for people to master language in their life. The language development of children at the age of 3 or 4 is largely dependent on external environmental stimuli and depends on the influence education. It is an important prereguisite to create a family-style warm, loose and free language environment for children to develop their language.

3-4 years old is the most critical period for children's language development, and it is a arduous task to improve children's language expression ability. In education, we must create a rich and colorful living environment for children and give them a free family-style language atmosphere. The use of literary works to cultivate children's good early reading habits is an important educational method. In a warm, relaxed and free language environment, children can develop their abilities and interests in all aspects of language better.

5.2.2　Characteristics of attention development

4-year-old children can be strengthened through training, and the following points should be paid attention to in early childhood teaching.

5.2.2.1　Defining the purpose of learning

The clearer the children's purpose of learning, the easier it is to sustain their attention.

5.2.2.2　Cultivate interest

When children are interested in a certain content, their attention is easy to focus and last, so the forms of early childhood education should be diversified and vivid.

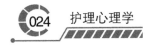

5.2.2.3　Create a good environment for learning

When studying, try to keep indoor and outdoor quiet, adults don't walk around the house, don't children speak irrelevant to the content of the study.

5.2.3　Characteristics of imagination development

4-year-old children's imagination is generally poor and simple, lacking a clear purpose, mainly involuntary imagination, intentional imagination and creative imagination are gradually developing, but not dominant. Unintentional imagination main features.

5.2.3.1　Imaginative themes

The imaginary themes are changeable and can not go on for a certain purpose, and it is easy to move from one theme to another. For example, one day I want to be a doctor, and another day I want to be a policeman.

5.2.3.2　Imagination and reality are indistinguishable

Imagination is inseparable from reality, and can not clearly distinguish imagined things from real things. Therefore, it is often mistaken for a lie. For example, he likes car toys, and he imagines other children's cars as his own, saying that this car is mine.

5.2.3.3　Imagination has a special exaggeration

Likes to exaggerate certain features or plots of things. For example, ask a child how tall you want to be, and he will answer "as tall as the sky".

5.2.4　Development of thinking

Piaget believes that the thinking of children aged 2-7 belongs to the preoperational stage, which is the period when children overcome various psychological obstacles and gradually transition to logical thinking. At this stage, children are mainly expressive thinking, and the basic characteristics of thinking are relative specificity, irreversibility, egocentricity and rigidity.

Section 3　Psychological Development of Preschool Children

5.3.1　Active conflict with guilt

During this period, if the active inquiry behavior shown by the young child is encouraged, the young child will form the initiative, which will lay the foundation for him to become a responsible and creative person in the future. If adults laugh at young children's original behavior and imagination, young children will gradually lose self-confidence, which makes them more inclined to live in a narrow circle arranged for them by others, and lack the initiative to create a happy life by themselves.

When children's sense of initiative outweighs their sense of guilt, they have the quality of "purpose". Erickson defines purpose as: "A courage to face and pursue worthy goals that is not limited by the young child's imagined fear of failure, guilt, and punishment."

5.3.2   Development of self-awareness

Under the influence of education, children's self - awareness has further developed. Relevant studies have shown that the general trend of the development of various factors of children's self-awareness is to increase with age.

5.3.2.1   Development of self-concept

Before the age of seven, children's self - description is limited to physical characteristics, age, genderand favorite activities, and does not describe internal psychological characteristics. Early cognitive ability of children is in the stage ofconcrete image thinking, they are easy to confuse self, body and mind. The concept of children is "physical concept", children do notdistinguish between internal psychological experience and external physical experience.

5.3.2.2   Development of self-evaluation

The ability of self - evaluation is not obvious in 3 - year - old children. The turning age of self - evaluation is 3. 5-4. 0 years old, and the development speed of this age is faster than that of 4-5 years old. Most 5-year-old children have been able to conduct self-evaluation.

The characteristics of children's self-evaluation are as follows.

(1) From trusting adult evaluation to independent evaluation.

(2) From the evaluation of external behavior to the evaluation of inner qualities.

(3) From a more general evaluation to a more detailed evaluation.

In general, children's self-evaluation ability is still very poor, adult evaluation of childrens personality development plays a developmental role. Therefore adults must be good at making appropriate evaluations of children. It is harmful for children to make too high or too low an evaluation of their behavior.

Section 4   Emotional Development of Preschool Children

5.4.1   Rapid development of empathy

Children aged 4-5 have strong empathy ability, they can put themselves in other people's situation, put themselves in other people's shoes, and accept other people's emotions. Empathic young children are more likely to transform empathy arousal into concern for the grieving person, which ultimately promotes the development of altruistic behavior. For example, when a child sees a companion lose a fun toy due to damage. When he was sad, he would think: if he lost such a toy, he would be sad too. Sadness at this time is an egocentric transference that shifts the situation of the partner onto oneself. At the same time he will also think that he is my companion, he is sad, so I am sad too, and should help and comfort him. In addition, due to the development of language, children aged 4-5 have learned more emotional words, such as happy, afraid, uncomfortable, angry, like, hate, love, boring. They often use these emotional words to describe themselves and others. They can also use a variety of emotional language to appease others or influence their behavior.

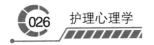

5.4.2 Emotional understanding depends on social knowledge

The age of 4–5 is a critical period for the development of children's emotional understanding ability. At this stage, children's understanding of emotions is in the stage of social knowledge dependence, and they are more inclined to make stereotyped speculations about other people's emotions and make corresponding behavioral responses based on their own social knowledge. Children aged 4–5 can applysocial behavioral norms and initially evaluate their own behavior. They can also regulate their own behavior with the help of adults. Self-control ability begins to form, and they have a preliminary sense of responsibility and morality. Children's interpersonal relationships have also undergone major changes, transitioning to peer relationships, being able to cooperate friendly and to experience their own inner psychological activities. However, young children in this matter are still more self-centered in terms of cognition and emotion, and are prone to infer the emotions of others based on their own thoughts, and their ability to recognize and manage other people's emotions is weak.

Section 5   Health Assessment and Nursing of Preschool Children

Preschool children's range of activities is expanded, their intelligence develops rapidly, their self-care ability is enhanced, and their body resistance is gradually enhanced, but they are still susceptible to childhood infectious diseases. The focus of health care is continue to monitor growth and development; strengthen early education, cultivate independent living ability and good moral quality; strengthen physical exercise to enhance physical fitness; prevent infectious diseases and prevent accidents. Strengthen the management of kindergarten institutions.

The specific measures for health care are as follows.

5.5.1   Nutrition

The diet of preschool children is close to that of adults, with three meals a day and 2–3 snacks. Children's appetite is greatly affected by activities and emotions. Ways to increase appetite include allowing children to rest for a few minutes before eating, maintaining a pleasant and relaxed atmosphere during meals, using children's favorite utensils and comfortable tables and chairs. Adults should model healthy eating habits and good dining etiquette for children. Preschool children like to participate in food preparation and table setting. Parents can take advantage of this opportunity to conduct health education on nutrition knowledge, food hygiene and scalding prevention.

5.5.2   Daily activities

Preschool children already have the ability to take care of themselves. When they learn self-care behaviors such as eating, washing face, brushing teeth, although their movements are slow and uncoordinated, they often need help from others, which may cost adults more time and energy. But children should be encouraged to make them more independent. Preschool children sleep 11–12 h a day. During this period, children's imagination is extremely rich, so they often have the phenomenon of being afraid of the dark and having nightmares at night. Parents who need to appease their children can turn on a small light indoors. Before going to bed, you can do some relaxing and pleasant activities with your child to reduce tension. Preschoolers are very active and get more exercise from daily play and activities. Health personnel should also guide parents to make full use of air, sunlight and water during physical exercise in children, and carry out three-bath exercise.

5.5.3   To protect the teeth

Pay attention to deciduous tooth caries. Improper cleaning of teeth during the period can lead to caries in primary teeth, and if not treated in time, it will seriously affect the growth of permanent teeth. When double teeth appear, deciduous teeth should be extracted, otherwise the teeth will be misaligned and the bite will be misaligned. balanced diet. A diet that is too refined can lead to decreased chewing function of teeth and poor jaw development. Children should be guaranteed a balanced nutrition. Get your child to break bad habits like licking their teeth. Bad habits such as licking your teeth can cause deformities such as irregular dentition, affecting the function of the teeth and the appearance of the face. Oral cleaning should be done well. Special attention should be paid to the maintenance of teeth, keep the mouth clean, insist on brushing your teeth in the morning and evening, and rinse your mouth after meals.

Chapter 6 Development of School-age Children

Summary

Objectives

1. Master primary school child care work.
2. Understand the characteristics of primary school children's psychological, cognitive, social and emotional development.
3. Understand the characteristics of the physical development of primary school children.

Age 7-13 is the period when children begin to enter primary school. This is an important turning point in children's psychological development. In the lower grades of primary school, children also have obvious psychological characteristics of preschool children, while children in the upper grades of primary school gradually enter puberty with the change of physical age. For this reason, the elementary years are often referred to as the prepubertal period.

The psychology of primary school students is in a period of rapid and coordinated development. The primary school stage is a good time to promote intellectual development, form a harmonious personality, and cultivate good psychological quality and behavioral habits.

Section 1 Physiological Development of School-age Children

The brain structure of primary school students has developed rapidly, and the 12-year-old child is 1,400 g, reaching the level of adults. 7-year-old slept an average of 11 h, 10-year-old 10 h, and 12-year-old 9-10 h. After the age of 12, the child's intellectual development is basically finalized. The lower grade students are generally 6-8 years old and are in a period of steady development physiologically. Skeletal muscles thrive, especially the bones of the lower extremities, faster than the body. However, the muscles are not fully developed, the water content is high, the muscle fibers are thin, the tendons are wide and short, the cartilage of the joints is thick, the capsular ligaments are thin and loose, the muscles around the joints are slender, and the joints have a wider range of extension activities, the firmness is poor, and it is prone to dislocation. At the same time, the blood circulation is faster and the heartbeat is faster, which should prevent the heart from being overburdened and excessive physical activity. The coordination of large muscle movements is greatly developed than in childhood, but the coordination of small muscle movements is still poor. For example, first-year students are not only slow but also untidy when writing. Children at this stage are not easy to do sports with too much intensity and too long. When training small muscle movements such as writing and playing the piano, attention should be paid to the standardization of the movements.

Generally speaking, the physical development is in a relatively stable stage. In addition to the brain, the physiological indicators of the students in the third and fourth grade are only improved in quantity compared with the students in the first and second grade. Basically, there is no qualitative leap and they are still in a period of stable development. The physical performance of male and female students is obvious, and the female students are earlier than the male students. The moisture content of the muscles of the third and fourth grade students is higher, and the muscles are slender and tender. The ratio of heart volume to blood vessel volume in third and fourth graders is smaller than that in seniors. The nervous system of the third and fourth grade students develops rapidly, and the function of excitement and inhibition is enhanced. The average time for students to sleep every day is about 10 h, the waking time is increased, and the ability to control and regulate their own behavior is improved significantly.

Grade 5 and 6 students are generally 10 – 12 years old, which belongs to the juvenile period of human development. Generally speaking, the body development is in the peak growth stage. The physical fitness index of students in grade 5 and 6 has been improved. The male students are better than the female students in sprinting. The development of agility is also very sensitive, and the students learn and master technical movements quickly. The heart of grade five or six students still belongs to the characteristics of primary school students, pulse frequency is faster, but the heart development is very significant, has been close to the characteristics of middle school puberty. Therefore, appropriately increasing the amount of exercise will make students' heart volume and heart function develop significantly. The weight of 11 – 12 year old students' brains is close to the level of adults, and the function of brain activity has been significantly improved, and the function of brain stimulation has also been enhanced. 11 – 12 year old students can sleep an average of 9 hours. Fifth and sixth grade students, physical development again into a period of rapid development, known as the second development period. Not only do they gain height and weight significantly, but their musculoskeletal strength rapidly increases, especially by the sixth grade, when secondary sexual characteristics begin to appear.

Section 2   Elementary School-age Children's Psychological Development

6.2.1   Conflict of diligence and inferiority

Children at this stage should be educated in school. Schools are places where children are trained to adapt to society and acquire the knowledge and skills necessary for life in the future. If they can successfully complete the course of study, they will gain a sense of diligence, which gives them confidence in living independently and taking on work tasks in the future. On the contrary, there will be low self-esteem. Moreover, the life of a child who develops attitudes that place too much value on his own work, while ignoring others, is a miserable life. "If he sees his job as his only task and what he does as his only value, he may be the most tame and thoughtless slave of his job skills and of his bosses." Erickson said.

When children's sense of diligence is greater than their sense of inferiority, they acquire the quality of "ability". "Competence is not diminished by a child's inferiority complex", Erickson said, "What is required to accomplish a task is the proficiency and wisdom of free operation."

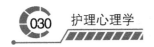

6.2.2 Cognitive development of school-age children

6.2.2.1 Development of school-age children's thinking ability

(1)Generalizing ability development

This development is manifested in that children can develop from the generalization of the external characteristics of things (image generalization) to the generalization of the essential attributes of things (abstract generalization); from the generalization of simple things to the generalization of complex things. The generalization ability of primary school children develops gradually with age, but the process of development is sometimes fast and sometimes slow, and the cognitive development of different tasks is not synchronized.

(2)Comparative competency development

From the difference between things to the same point of comparison, from the similarities and differences of concrete things to the similarities and differences of abstract things, from the intuitive comparison to the use of words and comparison in themind. Research shows that the development of primary school children's comparative ability is manifested in from distinguishing the similarities and differences of specific things, gradually developing to distinguishing the similarities and differences of many partial relationships; gradually developing from the comparison under the condition of direct perception to the condition of using language to cause images in the mind. The comparisons of elementary school children are not the same in all conditions, comparing some things to find both similarities and subtle differences, but in other conditions they compare differently.

6.2.2.2 Learning characteristics of school-age children

(1)Learning is the leading activity for primary school children

School learning is a purposeful and systematic acquisition of knowledge, skills and behavioral norms under the guidance of teachers. In this special learning process, children acquire knowledge, skills, and master a sense of social responsibility and obligation.

(2)Teaching and learning are two-way interactions between teachers and students

Teachers' teaching is to answer questions, solve doubts, and educate people in the process of imparting knowledge. Students are active learners and should not be regarded as passive recipients. Teaching and learning is a process of active interaction between teachers and students.

6.2.2.3 Characteristics of social development of school-age children

Sociality is the sum of all characteristics and typical behaviors that are compatible with social existence, developed in the process of individual socialization.

(1)Parent-child relationship

After children enter school, their relationship with their parents changes a lot. It is manifested as changes in the time, content and mode of communication between children and their parents. Compared with the preschool period, primary school children spend less time with their parents, parents pay less attention to children, and children's attachment and dependence on their parents are weakened. In terms of communication content, parents of primary school children pay more attention to their children's academics and morals. Such as tutoring, checking homework, discussing with the child what is happening at school, discussing the appropriateness of daily behavior. In terms of communication style, parental control begins to weaken in elementary school, and research shows that as children grow older, children make more and more decisions by themselves, and most things for children before the age of 6 are determined by parents.

(2) Peer communication and the formation of peer groups

Peer interaction is a unique way of socialization in which children form and develop personality traits and form social behaviors, values and attitudes. The main characteristics of peer interaction are more time with peers and more complex forms of interaction; enhanced skills in transmitting information in peer interaction, they can better understand the motives and purposes of others, and can better respond to others. Communication among their peers is more effective; they are better at using information to determine their actions toward others; better at coordinating interactions with his other children; beginning to form peer groups.

Section 3   Elementary School-age Children's Emotional and Personality Development

6.3.1   Emotional development of school-age children

With the gradual increase of age and the enrichment of life experience, the content of primary school children's emotions is constantly enriched, the emotions are further differentiated, and the methods of expressing emotions are also becoming more and more abundant. The depth of their emotions continues to increase, their ability to attribute things increases, and they tend to become more realistic. Emotional stability and controllability are significantly enhanced, and they are no longer as rushing as preschoolers. Elementary school children can gradually control their emotions. Moreover, at this stage, children's sense of morality and rationality gradually develops, and they are gradually able to make certain judgments about behavior, their curiosity is also stronger and stronger, and they have a wide range of interests in learning and life.

6.3.2   Character development of school-age children

The so-called character refers to the individual psychological characteristics manifested in the individual's stable attitude towards reality and the corresponding behavior style, which is mainly manifested in the individual's attitude toward reality and the individual behavior style. Children in primary school are in the period of character formation. Although children in this period have initially formed the ability to deal with things independently, they are still very easy to accept the influence of the social environment, especially the influence of the family. Because they are in the formative period of their character, the attitude characteristics of primary school children's characters are unstable and often sway from side to side. The intellectual characteristics of elementary school children are stable from the second to the fourth grade, and there is a period of rapid development from the fourth to the sixth grade. The emotional characteristics of elementary school children are constantly developing, and the intensity and persistence of emotions develop faster, because sixth-grade children are just entering adolescence, and their behaviors are particularly susceptible to emotional influence. From the perspective of character will, the self-control and

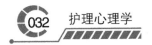

persistence of primary school children showed a downward trend. The reason is that children in lower grades are subject to external control. As they grow older, their dependence on external control decreases, but internal control has not yet developed and is not enough to regulate and control themselves.

Section 4   Physical and Mental Care of School-age Children

For primary school child care work, it is mainly carried out from two aspects: physical and psychological.

6.4.1   Physical care work

Primary school is a golden period for children's growth and development, and they need more nutrients. They can eat more nutritious foods to help children grow. For elementary school students, they need to eat more foods rich in protein, vitamins and calcium in order to meet the nutritional needs of the body and grow higher. For elementary school children, because they enter the learning stage, they need to develop a normal life and rest, so they should pay attention to children's breakfast and snacks between classes. Supplement milk, walnuts, fish and other substances. Milk is not only rich in protein and amino acids, but also contains a lot of calcium, phosphorus and other minerals. Not only is it beneficial to growth and development, but it is especially beneficial for the growth of the most critical bones. Walnuts have a lot of nutrients. They not only contain a lot of fatty acids, which can reduce the body's inflammatory response, prevent cardiovascular disease, and help control diabetes. The manganese contained in walnuts helps strengthen bones, and magnesium helps organs and muscles, the normal work of the nervous system. Fish is rich in vitamin B_1 necessary for the body, and there are many proteins that can enhance the body's resistance. Eating more fish can also help the brain's health and improve the body's memory.

6.4.2   Psychological care work

Primary school is not only the initial stage of basic education, but also a critical period for students to experience knowledge, acquire knowledge and master skills. During primary school, students must have the correct attitude towards learning, good study habits, etc., in order to lay a solid foundation for future study and life. However, when entering the early stage of primary school, due to the jumping changes, some students in the lower grades of primary school have a phenomenon of maladaptation in learning, which leads to problems such as a decline in students' academic performance and a lack of interest in learning. Stimulate learning interest and improve learning efficiency. Confucius said: "Those who know are not as good as those who are good, and those who are good are not as good as those who enjoy themselves." Interest in learning is the core element of maintaining a good attention ability, and it is also a powerful driving force for learning. Once students' interest in learning is stimulated, their learning efficiency will continue to increase. Lower primary school students are active, curious, imitative and malleable, and will be interested in novel things. Follow the age characteristics of students and teach students in accordance with their aptitude. Zhu Xi, a famous educator, once said: "Sages and sages teach according to their aptitudes. The small is the small, the big is the big, and no one is abandoned." Implementing teaching in accordance with aptitude requires teachers to proceed from reality and respect the existing physical and mental development of students. According to the situation, learn to promote the development of morality, intelligence, physique, aesthetics and labor in the lower grades of primary school from different perspectives. In the teaching process, teachers should not only implement education to all students, but also do not give up underachievers, and always seize the shining points of each student.

Chapter 7　Development of Adolescents

Summary

Objectives

1. Master the performance and development characteristics of adolescents' self – awareness, emotion, morality and interpersonal communication. Master the physical and mental care of young people.
2. Understand the general characteristics of adolescent personality and social development.
3. Understand the general characteristics of individual physical and mental development during adolescence.

Section 1　Physiological Development of Adolescent

Adolescence is a period of transition from childhood to adulthood. During this period, adolescents undergo tremendous physical and psychological changes. Adolescence is the peak period of individual physical development and sexual maturity. Physical maturity makes adolescents feel adult psychologically, they want to acquire certain rights as adults, find new standards of behavior and desire to change social roles. However, due to their limited level of psychological development, many expectations can not be fulfilled, and they are prone to frustration. In short, due to the unbalanced physical and mental development at this stage, young people are faced with various psychological crises and some psychological and behavioral problems.

The physical development of adolescence is mainly manifested in adolescence, and the sharp increase in height and weight of adolescents and the development of secondary sexual characteristics all occur in adolescence. After entering the early adolescence, the individual gradually reaches sexual maturity, and the adolescent's heart, lungs, brain and nervous system also continue to develop, and these physiological development processes are basically completed at the end of the early adolescence.

Adolescence is the second peak period of individual growth and development. During this period, the body and physiological functions of adolescents have undergone drastic changes, mainly in three aspects: changes in body shape, enhancement of internal functions, and sexual development and maturity. These are the three major changes in the physiological development of adolescence.

7.1.1　Changes in body shape

Adolescents have rapid physical development, and their height, weight and face have undergone great changes, and these changes have gradually made them closer to adults in appearance.

7.1.1.1   Growth in height

The most obvious feature of adolescent appearance changes is the rapid increase in height. There are two peaks in the growth of human height. The first peak occurs at about 1 year old, when the height generally increases by more than 50%; the second peak of growth occurs in adolescence. At this stage, the height of adolescents grows abnormally rapidly.

7.1.1.2   Weight gain

Adolescents during puberty also experience greater developmental changes in body weight. From the weight growth curve of urban and rural boys and girls in China, it can be seen that boys gain the fastest weight during the period of 12–14 years old, with an average annual increase of 5.0 kg. The growth peak is at the age of 13, and the growth rate decreases rapidly after the age of 15. Girls gain the fastest weight at age 11–13, gaining an average of 4.5 kg per year, peak growth at age 11–12, and decline rapidly after age 13.

7.1.1.3   The appearance of secondary sexual characteristics

Secondary sexual characteristics are the external manifestations of sexual development and are an important sign of changes in the body shape of adolescents. With the emergence of secondary sexual characteristics, adolescents begin to move from a neutral state of childhood to a state of gender differentiation. In men, secondary sexual characteristics are mainly manifested as a prominent Adam's apple, a low voice, a tall physique, well-developed muscles, beards on the lips, numerous and dense hairs around the body, and axillary and pubic hair. In women, secondary sexual characteristics are characterized by a thin voice, bulging breasts, a wide pelvis, more subcutaneous fat, enlarged buttocks, plump body, and the appearance of armpit and pubic hair. The appearance of these secondary sexual characteristics makes the difference in appearance between male and female adolescents increasingly obvious.

7.1.2   Enhancement of body functions

During puberty, various physiological functions in an individual grow rapidly and gradually reach maturity.

7.1.2.1   Enhancement of cardiac compressor performance

Some new functional features appeared in the cardiovascular system of adolescents. Morphologically, in order to meet the needs of the growth spurt in puberty, the cardiovascular system, which is the human transport system, also experienced a second growth acceleration. At age 9, a child's heart weight is 6 times that at birth, and after the onset of puberty, it increases to 12–14 times; similarly, heart density increases exponentially during puberty. And, due to the increased activity of adolescents, the muscles that make up the walls of the ventricles thicken and the fibers of the heart muscle become more elastic, creating conditions for the heart to squeeze more blood with each contraction. In terms of function, the main performance is that the heart rhythm and pulse begin to slow down. On the one hand, the nerve fibers that control the heart activity have been fully developed and can regulate the heart activity more effectively. It takes 70–80 beats to meet the body's needs.

7.1.2.2   Development of the lungs

During adolescence, lung development is also markedly accelerated. Around the age of 12, the weight of

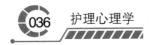

the lungs is 10 times that at birth, the structure of the pulmonary lobules is gradually improved, the capacity of the alveoli increases, and the development of certain muscles related to breathing is accelerated, which further strengthens the respiratory function. Throughout puberty, lung capacity will more than double that before puberty. There are significant differences in lung capacity between men and women.

7.1.2.3　Enhanced muscle strength

Weight gain in adolescent teens indicates changes in muscles and bones. There are also significant differences between men and women in the level of development of muscle strength.

7.1.2.4　Brain development

In terms of quantity, the growth of brain weight and brain volume in adolescents is not significant, because children's brain weight is 95% of that of adults before the age of 10. But in terms of quality, the development of the brain has made great progress at this time. Research on brain waves in China shows that individuals have two accelerated periods of brain development between the ages of 4 and 20, the first occurs at the age of 5−6, and the second occurs around the age of 13, that is, adolescence. The nervous system is basically no different from that of adults. The sulci and gyri of the cerebral cortex are well assembled, and the nerve fibers are myelinated. As the brain and nervous system mature, the excitement and inhibition of adolescents also tend to balance.

7.1.3　Sexual development and maturation

The reproductive system is the most mature of all systems in the human body, and its maturity marks the completion of the human body's physiological development.

7.1.3.1　Increased sex hormones

Sex hormone secretion is an important part of the activity of the entire endocrine system. Before puberty, both men and women secrete only a small amount of sex hormones. After entering puberty, the secretion of gonadotropin-releasing hormone in the individual's hypothalamus increases, so that the secretion of gonadotropin in the anterior pituitary also increases, which in turn leads to a corresponding increase in the level of gonadal hormones and promotes gonadal development. The female gonads are the ovaries and the male gonads are the testes. The maturation of the gonads causes menstruation in women and nocturnal emission in men.

7.1.3.2　Development of sexual organs

The female sex organs include the ovaries, uterus and vagina. Development is slow before puberty, accelerated at 8−10 years of age, and then skyrockets. The uterus develops from the age of 10 to the age of 18. The length has been doubled, and the shape and proportions of its parts have also changed.

Male sexual organs include testes, epididymis, seminal vesicles, prostate and penis. Men's sex organs develop later than women's, developing very slowly before the age of 10, and accelerating after puberty.

Section 2　Psychological Development of Adolescent

With a series of special changes in adolescents' physiology and intelligence, many new characteristics have emerged in their psychological development, which are manifested in many aspects such as self-awareness, emotions, daily mentality, and relationships with parents and peers. Generally speaking, there are two personality characteristics of adolescents: one is imbalance; the other is extreme or paranoid.

7.2.1   Development of self-awareness

7.2.1.1   Basic characteristics of self-awareness

Adolescence is the second leap in the development of self-awareness. Before an individual reaches adolescence, there is a leap in the development of self-awareness, between the ages of 1 and 3, and it is an important feature that children can use the pronoun "I" to identify themselves. In the next few years, although the child's self-awareness continued to develop, the rate of development was relatively steady.

After entering puberty, due to the rapid development of the body, adolescents quickly develop the physical features of adults. Because this kind of physiological change happened too suddenly, they felt a sense of panic, and at the same time, they consciously or unconsciously pulled back a large part of their thoughts from the objective world they had been playing in, and redirected them to subjective world makes the ideology enter the self again, which leads to the second leap of self-consciousness. The outstanding performance of the high self-awareness is that the inner world of the teenagers is becoming richer and richer, and they often usea lot of their minds for introspection in daily life and school. "What kind of person am I?" "What are my characteristics?" "Do other people like me or hate me?" A series of questions about "me" began to revolve in their minds repeatedly. It can often be clearly observed in compositions and diaries. For example, in the same composition with the content of "what did I see", primary school students purely describe the scene of the objective world, while teenagers still describe the objective world, but their descriptions have a strong personal emotional tone. In the composition, the personal preferences, troubles and longings are more prominent.

Another major manifestation of the heightened self-consciousness in adolescence is the subjective paranoia of its personality. On the one hand, they always think they are right and don't listen to other people's opinions, on the other hand, they feel that others always seem to treat them with a critical attitude. Therefore, when you hear others talking in a low voice, you will judge that you are talking about yourself; when you see others smiling, you will think that you are laughing at yourself; if a teacher takes one more look at yourself, you will think that you are doing something wrong...

7.2.1.2   Self-concept

Personality formation also includes having a relatively stable self-concept or self-image. Whether a person has an appropriate self-concept is crucial to the development of his personality.

The cognitive abilities of individuals in adolescence are greatly improved, and they can recognize themselves in more abstract, complex and unique ways, so the self-concept of adolescents is very different in content and structure from the self-concept of early individuals.

(1) Self-concept is more abstract

Piaget theorized that individuals transition from concrete operational thinking to formal operational thinking at the age of 11 or 12. Individuals entering adolescence have stopped describing their characteristicsin very specific terms (e. g. , "I like food") and more often in general terms (e. g. , "I am a

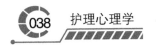

real person"). In early adolescence, the individual's self-concept is more abstract, focusing not only on personality traits, but also on important values and ideologies and beliefs (e. g., "I am a pseudo-liberal").

(2) Self-concept is more integrated and organized

When adolescents describe themselves, they not only list various aspects of the self as early children do, but also integrate their self-perceptions, including seemingly contradictory aspects, into a more logical and coherent unity.

(3) The structure of self-concept is more differentiated

Adolescents no longer use certain traits to describe themselves in general terms like childhood individuals, but instead recognize that the self behaves differently in different situations. For example, adolescents describe themselves by distinguishing between their parents, friends, peers, and lovers, and they also develop different self-concepts based on their different social roles.

7.2.1.3　Self-evaluation

Self-evaluation refers to an individual's evaluation of his own thoughts, abilities, levels, etc., and it is the main component of the self-regulation mechanism. The capacity for self-evaluation only begins to mature in early youth. Although individuals began to produce some simple self-evaluations in childhood, most of the self-evaluations at that time were produced by the reflection of others' attitudes and reactions to themselves, and lacked introspection. In the early stage of youth, due to the further development of abstract logical thinking and the increasing enrichment of knowledge and experience, young people gradually learn to view and analyze themselves more comprehensively, objectively and dialectically, and their ability to self-evaluate becomes comprehensive, active, and increasingly profound. It is mainly manifested in that they can not only analyze their temporary ideological contradictions and psychological states, but also recognize their individual psychological characteristics that dominate a specific behavior, and can often evaluate their entire psychological appearance, and recognize that they are relatively stable personality and psychological quality.

7.2.2　Characteristics of emotional development

The emotional performance of adolescents fully reflects the contradictory characteristics of semi-mature and semi-naive. With the development of adolescents' psychological ability and the expansion of life experience, their emotional feelings and expressions are no longer as simple as before, but they are far less stable than adults' emotional experience, showing a clear duality.

7.2.3　Characteristics of interpersonal communication

In the relationship with peers, there are obvious differences between adolescents and childhood children, mainly in the following aspects.

7.2.3.1　Gradually overcome the way gangs communicate

The most obvious feature of childhood friends in making friends is the phenomenon of gangs, which is manifested by 6 or 7 children who often interact and play together. In this interaction, they feel free and happy both physically and mentally. So, in terms of making friends, elementary school is the age of gangs. In the upper grades of elementary school, this gang form of making friends has developed to its peak, and then tends to disintegrate and be replaced by new forms of communication.

7.2.3.2 Friendships are increasingly important in teens' lives

Teens also have a new appreciation for what it means to make friends. They believe that friends should be able to share weal and woe, and be able to get support and help from each other. Therefore, they have special requirements for the quality of friends, believing that friends should be frank, reasonable, concerned about others, and keep secrets. In the daily interactions of teenagers, good friends often reveal to each other what they think is the most important and secret. This kind of communication is of positive significance to the psychological development of young people, which enables them to better understand their inner world and understand themselves better through others. This process has positive effects on the formation of self-concept, perspective-taking andidentity.

Consistency in views and actions is also one of the important conditions for psychological closeness among adolescent friends. On some occasions, good friends often have to work out a consistent course of action, and if they violate the course, they will be severely reprimanded. They believe that being faithful to agreements and friends is a very important measure of friendship.

Section 3   Cognitive Development of Adolescent

According to Piaget's stage theory of cognitive development, adolescents are in the stage of formal operational thinking (ages 11 and above). The main characteristic of thinking at this stage is that the form and content of things canbe separated in the mind, the specific things can be separated, and logical deductions can be made based on assumptions, and formal operations can be used to solve problems such as combination, inclusion, proportion, exclusion, probability and factors. Analysis and other logical topics.

Two stages of adolescence: adolescence and early adolescence. The image thinking of the individual in adolescence tends to mature, and the abstract logical thinking begins to prevail. From the second grade of junior high school, students' abstract logical thinking begins to transform from the empirical level to the theoretical level. Therefore, the basic feature of junior high school students' thinking activities is that abstract logical thinking has taken the lead, but sometimes the specific image elements in thinking still play a role. The image thinking of young individuals has fully developed and matured, and the development of abstract logical thinking has also entered a mature stage. By the second year of senior high school, the transformation from empirical to theoretical has been initially completed, marking the maturity of their abstract logical thinking. Therefore, the development of logical thinking is the focus of the development of young people's thinking.

Logical thinking can be divided into two categories: formal logical thinking and dialectical logical thinking according to the different logical laws followed and methods used in thinking. Formal logical thinking and dialectical logical thinking are two different development stages of abstract logical thinking. Dialectical logical thinking is based on formal logical thinking and higher than formal logical thinking. The development and maturity of these two forms of thinking is an important sign of the development and maturity of adolescent thinking. The development of formal logical thinking of senior high school students is relatively stable and uniform, while the development of dialectical logical thinking is relatively rapid. At this stage, its formal logic thinking has been quite perfect development, occupies a dominant position in thinking activities. However, the development level of dialectical logical thinking is lower than

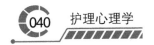

that of formal logical thinking, and the development of the two complement each other, making teenagers' thinking level higher, more mature and more perfect.

With the growth of age, the general trend of creative thinking level of teenagers is constantly moving forward, the higher the grade, the better the performance of creative thinking, but the development speed is uneven, the second year of high school is the high tide of creative thinking development, the first and third year of high school is the low tide of creative thinking development. With the increase of age, the fluency of creative thinking of senior high school students shows a declining trend, the flexibility is in stable development, and the uniqueness is gradually improved.

In addition to creative imagination and divergent thinking, the development of teenagers' creative thinking is also manifested in Epiphany, analogical transfer and hypothesis testing. The creative thinking of adolescents is at a high development stage, and the level of individual creative thinking has an important impact on the performance of their creativity.

Section 4   Physical and Mental Care of Adolescent

7.4.1   Psychological care

The arrangement of hospital beds should consider the age characteristics of adolescents as much as possible. Try to satisfy their lively and active nature, and provide them with appropriate space to create conditions so that they can be in a good mood and receive treatment with peace of mind during the hospitalization. Of course, it is also necessary to explain to them the relevant rules and regulations of the hospital as well as the knowledge and treatment methods of the disease, so that they can actively cooperate with the treatment.

Due to the developmental stage of puberty, the appearance of secondary physical characteristics often makes them particularly shy. They do not like the individual health guidance and physical examination conducted by medical staff of the opposite sex, but are more likely to accept the guidance of older and more mature doctors and nurses. Eager to know about their illness, but sometimes pretending to be uninterested and ashamed to talk about it, these are all related to the psychological characteristics of teenagers themselves, and in fact, it is a cover up by enterprising psychology for the psychology of wanting to know about the illness. Therefore, the protector should understand this point and take the initiative to give them some explanations and introductions about the disease, which is very beneficial to the treatment.

7.4.2   Physical health care

7.4.2.1   Develop good living habits

Make reasonable arrangements for life, work and study, cultivate good hygiene habits, and pay attention to physical exercise and proper labor. Personal hygiene includes oral hygiene, eye hygiene and proper posture for writing, reading, standing and sitting to prevent tooth decay, myopia and spinal curvature. The exercise content is systematically arranged according to different ages, and progresses in order.

7.4.2.2   Guaranteed sleep

Adequate sleep: adolescence sleep time 7−9 h, to develop good sleep habits.

7.4.2.3   Breast care

When a girl reaches puberty, her breasts will bulge, she should wear a bra in time, but the bra should not be too tight or too loose. Too tight will affect the normal development of the breasts, and too loose will not prevent the breasts from sagging.

Chapter 8 Development of Individuals in Early and Middle Adulthood

Summary

Objectives

1. Understand the basic issues of individual development in adulthood.
2. Understand the physical, psychological and cognitive changes at each stage of development.
3. Assess the need to meet individual health activity needs in adulthood.

Section 1 Overview for Individual in Early Adulthood

8.1.1 Age limit for early adulthood

The physical maturity of an individual is from 11 years old to 19 years old, that is, before the age of 20, when the physiology reaches full maturity. Thus, in a biological sense, the individual begins to enter early adulthood. Here we define the time of physical maturity as the onset age of early adulthood (the upper limit of early adulthood) and the maturity of social life as the end of early adulthood, which is the age of onset of mid- adulthood (the lower limit of early adulthood), according to which the age stage of early adulthood is defined as 19-40 years old.

8.1.2 General characteristics of early adulthood

Early adulthood is of great significance in the development of a person's life. During this period, the individual's physical and mental development tends to be stable and mature, the intellectual development reaches its heyday, a family is established, a career is established, and it begins to fully adapt to social life. Individuals in this period have the following characteristics.

8.1.2.1 Changes from the growth period to the stable period

The stage of childhood and adolescence is called the growth stage. The physical development of adolescence has reached a peak, and the psychology also tends to be initially mature. After entering early adulthood, individuals enter a stable phase. This kind of stability is reflected in the vast majority of individuals in their early adulthood, which are embodied as physiological development tends to be stable; psychological development, especially emotional process, tends to mature, and character characteristics are basically stereotyped; the way of life tends to be fixed and habitual; a relatively stable family has been established; the social occupation is stable, and they can be loyal to their duties.

8.1.2.2   Intellectual development reaches its heyday

The intellectual development of an individual in early adulthood is at its peak. The way of thinking has changed from formal logic thinking to dialectical logic thinking, and thinking is more relativity, flexibility, integration and practicality. In the final stages of early adulthood, the individual's creative thinking development also peaks and begins to show varying degrees of creativity in different domains.

8.1.3   Cognitive characteristics of early adulthood

8.1.3.1   Intellectual development in early adulthood

Intellectual development is an adaptive process. One of the important factors affecting the development of intelligence in early adulthood is the new objective environment in which the individual lives and the new adaptation tasks he faces.

Before the age of 18 or 19, the main task of an individual is to acquire a knowledge system related to social culture in order to eliminate contradictions with society, achieve adaptation to society, and realize socialization. The objective environment that the individual is in at this time is protected by adults. After entering early adulthood, after further formal or informal learning, individuals have basically mastered the cultural system and social moral system of their own nation, and have been able to adapt to the basic requirements of society, but at this time they are faced with new challenges in social life. Challenges, such as career, marriage, family, need to continue to conduct appropriate analysis, judgment, reasoning, to solve the problem.

8.1.3.2   General characteristics of intelligence in early adulthood

The overall level of intelligence performance in early adulthood shows relatively stable characteristics. At the same time, however, the intelligence of individuals in early adulthood exhibits qualitatively new properties. For example, individuals are in the knowledge acquisition stage during childhood and adolescence. Early adulthood is in the realization phase, where individuals must adapt their cognitive abilities to complex environments(such as marriage and work) in order to achieve long-term goals. At this stage individuals reduce knowledge acquisition activities and focus more on applying the acquired knowledge in daily life. Middle adulthood is in the stage of responsibility, which corresponds to fulfilling obligations and responsibilities. Old age is a period of recombination of knowledge.

8.1.3.3   Characteristics of memory development in early adulthood

In terms of memory, for individuals in early adulthood, although the mechanical memory ability has declined, the previous stage of early adulthood is the peak period of the development of logical memory ability in life. Intentional memory, understanding memory dominates, and the capacity of memory is also great.

8.1.3.4   Characteristics of imaginative development in early adulthood

In terms of imagination, the rational and creative elements in the individual's imagination in early adulthood have increased significantly, overcoming the illusory nature of the imagination in the previous developmental stages, and making the imagination more practical.

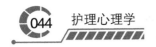

Section 2　Overview for Individual in Middle Adulthood

Middle adulthood, or middle age, generally refers to the period of the ages 40 – 65. The age range in mid – adulthood is relative, not set in stone. This is because with the improvement of living and medical conditions. The average life expectancy of people is increasing, and the age boundaries for young, middle – aged and old are also changing. Due to differences in individual cultivation and other aspects, even if the age is the same, the health status and the degree of aging may vary greatly.

As a stage in the life course, an individual in mid – adulthood undergoes a series of changes, both physiologically and psychologically. Because individuals in mid–adulthood face various tasks in the family and society and play various roles, and their development is affected by various variables, it is difficult to draw a unified conclusion on the research on the psychological characteristics of the center of adulthood. Mid–adulthood is also the current less studied age groups.

Middle – aged people are the backbone of society, the core of the family, and the main creators of material and spiritual wealth. Therefore, the family life and professional activities of middle–aged people are more important than other stages of the life course.

In the development of an individual's life course, the family is an important influencing factor throughout. Individuals are affected by this microenvironment, and at the same time have an impact on this microenvironment.

Like individual life, family also has a process of generation, development and extinction, and it presents certain periodic characteristics. The so – called family life cycle usually refers to the family development process that starts from the marriage between a man and a woman to form a family and ends with the death of both husband and wife leading to the disintegration of the family. The family life cycle is generally divided into several stages according to changes in the composition of family members and developmental tasks. At each stage, there are corresponding developmental issues that family members need to face or solve. How to face or solve these development issues is related to the psychological development process and life adaptation level of family members.

Section 3　Individual Care and Wellness Planning for Early and Middle Adulthood

8.3.1　Individual psychological care

In adulthood, due to the heavy burden and difficulties of domestic work, the emotions are often in a state of tension. Mental health during this period is very important.

8.3.1.1　Coordinate all aspects of interpersonal relationships

Strengthen self–control, be sincere and friendly in communication, avoid non–principled disputes, be strict with yourself, be generous with others, and have a good interpersonal relationship. Promote style for life and work.

8.3.1.2   Family harmony , marital harmony

Both personal and physical health. The foundation of a happy and happy life is also a strong guarantee of career success.

8.3.1.3   self-motivation

Through self-motivation , promoting the desire for achievement in career is the mainstream of adult psychological activities. The happiness of personal life is the auxiliary of career success , and striving for career success is the meaning of life.

8.3.2   Individual body care

8.3.2.1   Guaranteed sleep

First of all , develop good work and rest habits , create a good sleep environment , develop a good habit of falling asleep and getting up on time , stable sleep , and avoid causing excessive fatigue of cerebral cortex cells. The temperature in the bedroom is moderate , and some mild colors are used in the room , which can make the mood relaxed and suitable for sleep. Mental relaxation and stress relief. Relieve your own stress , such as through moderate exercise before going to bed , listening to music , and head massage to relieve stress. Take a short walk before going to bed , play soft and soothing music such as serenade while sleeping , use massage therapy , massage the head , face , behind the ears , neck and other parts before going to bed , all of which can relieve the fatigue of the whole body and promote sleep.

8.3.2.2   Healthy diet

The daily intake of young people is mainly cereal crops , and eggs , meat , and beans are abundant. Men's intake of vegetables , fruits , and dairy intake is relatively low ; women's intake of beans , fish and shrimp is relatively low. From the perspective of energy sources , fat accounts for a large proportion. Due to a large intake of fat , young people prematurely lead to high blood pressure , coronary heart disease and other sub-health diseases. In addition , young people's low intake of fruits and vegetables leads to vitamin and mineral deficiencies in the body , which seriously affects metabolism. Therefore , in the choice of foods , cereals , meat , dairy , vegetables and fruits should be included. Usually pay attention to the combination of food to ensure its nutritional balance.

8.3.2.3   Exercise

Exercising every day can help relieve work fatigue , improve resistance , move joints , improve body metabolism , and promote blood circulation. It can prevent three highs and is very beneficial to physical health.

Aerobic exercise is the most common and effective form of exercise for adults. During moderate-intensity aerobic exercise , the exercise intensity can be controlled within the range of 60% - 70% of the maximum heart rate , or equivalent to subjective physical strength level 12 - 14 : during high-intensity aerobic exercise , the exercise intensity can be controlled. Within the 70% - 80% maximum heart rate range , or equivalent to a subjective physical strength level of 15 - 16. Adults can use the following three ways to do aerobic exercise. Moderate-intensity aerobic exercise. Do 150 minutes or more of moderate-intensity aerobic activity per week for 30 minutes or more per day , 5 days per week. High-intensity aerobic exercise. Do more than 75 minutes of vigorous-intensity aerobic exercise every week. Exercise 25 minutes or more a day , 3 days a week. Textual aerobic exercise. Alternately perform moderate-intensity and high-

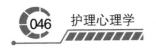

intensity aerobic exercise every week, such as 30 minutes or more of moderate-intensity aerobic exercise every Monday, Wednesday, and Friday, and 25 minutes or more of high-intensity aerobic exercise every Tuesday and Sunday.

For people with good physical function and good exercise habits, if they do 300 minutes of moderate-intensity aerobic exercise or 150 minutes of high-intensity aerobic exercise every week, the fitness effect is more obvious. It can not only enhance physical fitness, prevent and treat chronic diseases such as high blood pressure, dyslipidemia, and diabetes, but also effectively improve the immune function of the body. It also has a positive effect on preventing breast cancer, colon cancer and other chronic diseases. For adults who control or lose weight, 60 minutes of aerobic exercise a day can control weight gain, and more than 90 minutes of aerobic exercise a day can reduce body fat content and make weight loss. If you exercise at the same time, with the control of diet, the effect of weight loss is more obvious.

Chapter 9 Development of Individuals in Late Adulthood

Summary

Objectives

1. Master the challenges, developmental tasks, major mental health problems and general psychological characteristics in late adulthood.
2. Understand the general trends or characteristics of cognitive, emotional, personality and social development and changes in late adulthood.
3. Identify activities suitable for the elderly to meet the needs of the elderly.

Late adulthood, also known as late adulthood and old age, generally refers to the period from the age of 65 to decline. The basic characteristics of individual physical and mental changes in late adulthood are although individual differences are very large, the general trend is to gradually show degenerative changes.

Section 1　Cognitive Characteristics of Late Adulthood

9.1.1　Significant degenerative changes in perception

9.1.1.1　Visual impairment

With age, because the elasticity of the eye lens becomes smaller and the accommodation power gradually declines, it is often difficult to see close objects, and presbyopia occurs. Before the age of 45, the vision loss is relatively slow, and the decline accelerates after the age of 45. Reading glasses are generally required after the age of 45.

9.1.1.2　Hearing loss

Compared with vision, older people are more likely to have hearing deficits. According to statistics, among the 65–74 years old in the United States, 13% have hearing impairment; among the 75 years old, 26% have hearing impairment. A survey in our country found that 63.6% of the elderly suffer from hearing loss, and the hearing loss for high pitches is more obvious. Some people have hearing loss to the extent of deafness. Studies have pointed out that the optimal age of human hearing is 20 years old, and it will gradually decline after that. After the age of 30, the hearing threshold gradually increases with age. Beasley's research pointed out that people generally over the age of 50 hearing loss. The researchers believe that 50–59 years old can be regarded as the turning point of Chinese hearing aging. Language and hearing comprehension gradually declined with age, starting to decline significantly in the 70–79 years old group, especially in the 80–89 years old and over 90 years old. Therefore, when speaking to the elderly, the

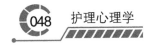

key parts should be slower and repeated several times; at the same time, do not change the topic suddenly, but look at the object, so that the elderly can judge the words by observing the movement of the speaker's lips.

9.1.1.3　Dullness of taste

Since taste receptors, taste buds, decrease with age, taste sensitivity also decreases with age. Studies have pointed out that people's sense of taste generally does not see much change before the age of 50, and after the age of 50, the stimulation threshold of taste increases. The diversity of taste also declines with age. Young people can taste multiple tastes in food at the same time, while older people often only feel a few of them. They are more sensitive to salty than others.

9.1.2　Memory declines with age

In daily life, people can often hear some complaints: "I am old, my memory is bad, and I often lose things." What is the relationship between people's memory and age? Does memory really decline in old age? What is the internal mechanism or cause of the recession?

Some psychologists have summarized the relationship between memory and age based on experimental research on memory: children's memory develops with age, and reaches its peak in adulthood. 18 - 30 years old is the "golden period" of human memory, and the efficiency of memory is the highest. After the age of 35, the trend of progressive decline in memory decline is assuming a 100% (highest) average memory score at 18 - 35 years old, then the average memory score is 95% at 35 - 60 years old, and 80% - 85% at 60 - 85 years old. Our country's research materials point out that people's memory has a relatively obvious decline stage after the age of 40, and then maintains a relatively stable level, until there is a more obvious decline stage after the age of 70. It can be seen that for most elderly people, the general trend of their memory changes is to decrease with age, mainly manifested as mechanical memory loss, memory span becomes smaller, speed memory performance within a specified time decline, recognition ability is poor, recall ability was significantly reduced, etc.

9.1.3　Changes in thinking

Some psychologists' research on the age difference of thinking shows that the efficiency of thinking processes such as concept learning and problem solving shows a gradual decline trend in old age. However, because thinking is an advanced and complex cognitive activity, research in this area has been slow. Until now, people still know little about the aging changes of thinking, and there are still different views on many issues. From a real-life perspective, government officials and decision makers in large and medium-sized enterprises are mainly those in their 50s, 60s or even over 70 years old, which shows that they still have high thinking ability. However, the results of the laboratory research show that the problem-solving ability of the elderly shows a general downward trend; when the decline begins, and the magnitude of the final decline, the conclusions of the studies are also inconsistent.

Section 2　Emotional Characteristics in Late Adulthood

The characteristics and influencing factors of emotion and emotion in late adulthood are not only a topic of concern to developmental psychologists, but also a practical issue related to the physical and mental health and quality of life of the elderly.

9.2.1　It is easier to have negative emotions

When a person reaches old age, due to the degenerative changes in physiology and psychology, as well as changes in role status and social interaction after retirement, it is easier to produce negative emotions such as depression, loneliness, aging and inferiority complex. Some domestic survey data illustrate this feature. A survey of 164 retirees in Shanghai showed that about 40% sometimes felt depression(including anxiety), 21.3% sometimes felt lonely, and 13.1% often felt lonely. A survey of 53 retired cadres in Beijing pointed out that 42% had no depression at all, 22% and 34% had slight and general depression respectively, and 2% had severe depression; 47% feel loneliness, 23% are slightly and generally. The feeling of middle use is similar, with slightly, generally and heavier accounting for 53%, 32% and 2%, respectively. Although we can not draw conclusions about the current emotions of the elderly in our country based on these preliminary surveys, these survey results at least give us the impression that the elderly in our country have a considerable number of various negative emotions.

9.2.2　Deep and lasting emotional experience

The emotional experience of the elderly is more profound. This is mainly reflected in their moral sense and aesthetic sense. In a questionnaire about moral sense, one question asked the subjects to choose "what do you think is the most important basic morality?" And the percentages who chose "love the motherland" were as follows: 18-30 years old accounted for 27.9%; 31-45 years old accounted for 38.3%; 46-60 years old accounted for 45.5%; over 60 years old accounted for 52.1%. It can be seen that the proportion of the elderly who regard "love of the motherland" as the most important basic morality is the highest among all age groups. When asked "What would you do if the municipal government issued a new policy on people's life and you have different opinions on it?", there are two age groups above 45 years old (i. e., middle - aged and elderly group), nearly half of the people chose to "report to government departments through various channels", while the number of people under the age of 45 who made this choice was greatly reduced. When asked "how will the political environment of our country change in the next 5 years?"The percentage of people under the age of 45 who answered "unsure" was significantly higher than that of middle-aged people over the age of 45. This shows that most of the elderly in our country are still full of political enthusiasm for the motherland and society, and have a high sense of responsibility.

Section 3　Nursing Work in Late Adulthood

With the progress of society and the development of medical technology, the average life expectancy in our country is increasing year by year, and the aging of the population has become a common problem faced by the medical profession and even the whole society. Improving the quality of life of the elderly is an important task for us at this stage. Now the common health problems and nursing care measures of the elderly are analyzed and sorted out as follows.

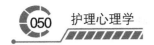

9.3.1　Common health problems in late adulthood

9.3.1.1　Retirement discomfort syndrome

The social status, economic status, and living environment of the elderly have changed due to retirement, and their activity space and work and rest rules have also changed. With normal communication and dialogue with young people, this huge gap often leads to physical and psychological discomfort, such as a sense of emptiness, uselessness, loneliness, and a sense of abandonment. It leads to depression and suicidal tendencies in some elderly people.

9.3.1.2　Various chronic diseases

With the improvement of living conditions, pollution of the ecological environment, bad eating habits, unreasonable dietary structure, the incidence of chronic diseases in the elderly is increasing year by year. At present, the most common chronic diseases of the elderly are hypertension, coronary heart disease, diabetes, stroke, malignant tumor, cerebellar degeneration syndrome, Parkinson syndrome, chronic bronchitis, etc., which greatly affect the quality of life of the elderly.

9.3.1.3　Empty nest effect

After the children grow up, due to various reasons, they can no longer live with their parents, and because they are busy with work or studies, they can not go home to visit their parents often, and communicate with their parents less and less, based on attachment and reluctance to the children, and worrying about their children outside often makes the elderly in the negative emotions of anticipation, worry, and worry all day long, which is extremely detrimental to the health of the elderly.

9.3.2　Nursing and health care measures in late adulthood

9.3.2.1　Guiding the elderly to self-care

Improve the awareness of preventing self-care defects: through health education for the elderly, make them realize that self-care has the same social value as helping others, so that they can voluntarily overcome and prevent self-care defects in life. Cultivate the ability of self-observation and judgment: through health education, the elderly can understand their own health status by looking, listening, smelling and touching. Once abnormality or early symptoms of disease are found, they should go to the hospital for medical treatment in time, and actively seek medical personnel's advice. Help to avoid delays in diagnosis and treatment.

9.3.2.2　Create a good home environment

Instruct the elderly to create a comfortable living environment: the room should be well lit, ventilated 2-3 times a day, the ventilation time should be about 30 minutes, the room temperature is suitable, and the temperature should be kept at 26-28 ℃ in summer and 20-22 ℃ in winter. , the humidity is kept at about 50%; at the same time, keep the ground flat and non-slip.

9.3.2.3　Reasonable diet

The dietary principles of the elderly are as follows. ①The food should be matched in thickness and size, which is conducive to digestion. ②Participate in regular physical activity to maintain energy balance. Besides, it is necessary to prevent dehydration in the elderly, because the elderly are not sensitive to thirst, and they are already in a state of mild dehydration when they feel thirsty. Therefore, it is recommended and urged that the elderly drink no less than 2,000 mL of water every day.

9.3.2.4   Good sleep

Good sleep can enhance immunity and make people energetic. Therefore, for the elderly with decreased sleep quality, active intervention should be given. The measures are as follows. Life should be regular and good living habits should be developed. Maintain emotional stability and combine work and rest. Create a suitable sleeping environment: the bedroom has soft lighting, and you can listen to some relaxing light music before going to bed.

9.3.2.5   Safe medication

Most of the elderly suffer from a variety of chronic diseases, therefore, long-term repeated medication is required, and most of them are combined medication. When administering medication for the elderly, scientific principles of medication should be followed, the risk of medication should be minimized, and the safety and effectiveness of medication should be ensured. Therefore, when taking the medicine, you should pay attention to the following. ① The dosage should not be too large. ② Do not use too many types of medication. ③ Strictly follow the doctor's instructions. ④ Pay close attention to the reaction after taking the medicine. ⑤ Store and keep medicines according to the package insert. Drugs that are easily decomposed when exposed to light should be stored in the dark; drugs that need to be stored at low temperature should be placed in a refrigerator at a constant temperature to avoid reducing the efficacy of the drug.

Chapter 10   Learning

Objectives
1. Define what is learning in psychology.
2. Identify and understand early learning theories.

Section 1   Concept of Learning

10.1.1   Definition of learning

A permanent change in behavior that occurs as the result of a prior experience.

When a person learns anything, some part of the brain is physically changed to record what they have learned.

Check process of learning in Figure 10-1.

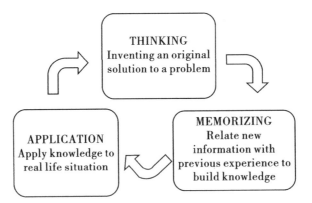

Figure 10-1   Process of learning

10.1.2   Learning of newborns

Newborn humans have almost no control of their muscles, except for their eyes and mouth. Imagine a baby born with complete control of all muscles, including arms, hands, legs, and feet. Would that be a good thing?

After the parents stopped bragging about their precocious youngster, they would discover what a nightmare they had. An infant with extreme mobility but no experience would get into every imaginable danger. From the start, people need to learn what is safe to touch and what isn't, where we can go and where we shouldn't. Just about everything we do requires constant learning and relearning.

Psychologists have devoted an enormous amount of research to learning, and in the process, they developed and refined research methods that they now routinely apply in other areas of psychological investigation. This chapter is about the procedures that change behavior—Why you lick your lips at the sight of tasty food? Why you turn away from a food that once made you sick? Why you handle sharp knives cautiously? And why you shudder if you see someone charging toward you with a knife?

Section 2 Learning Theories in the Early Stage

10.2.1 Classical conditioning

In the early 1900s, Ivan Petrovich Pavlov, a Russian physiologist who had won a Nobel Prize in Physiology or Medicine for his research on digestion, stumbled upon an observation that offered a simple explanation for learning. Given the rise of behaviorism, the mood of the time was ripe for Pavlov's ideas. One day as Pavlov was pursuing his digestion research, he noticed that adog secreted digestive juices as soon as it saw the lab worker who customarily fed the dogs. Because this secretion clearly depended on the dog's previous experiences, Pavlov called it a "psychological" secretion. he enlisted the help of other specialists, who discovered that "teasing" a dog with the sight of food produced salivation that was as predictable and automatic as any reflex. Pavlov called it a conditioned reflex because it depended on conditions.

Whenever Pavlov gave a dog food, the dog salivated. The food and salivation connection was automatic, requiring no training. Pavlov called food the unconditioned stimulus, and he called salivation the unconditioned response.

The unconditioned stimulus (UCS) is an event that automatically elicits an unconditioned response. The unconditioned response (UCR) is the action that the unconditioned stimulus elicits. Next Pavlov introduced a new stimulus, such as a metronome or other sound. Upon hearing the metronome, the dog lifted its ears and looked around but did not salivate, so the metronome was a neutral stimulus with regard to salivation. Pavlov sounded the metronome shortly before giving food to the dog. After a few pairings of the metronome with food, the dog began to salivate as soon as it heard the metronome.

We call the metronome the conditioned stimulus (CS), because a dog's response to it depends on the preceding conditions—that is, pairing the CS withthe UCS. The salivation that follows the metronomeis the conditioned response (CR). The conditioned response is whatever response the conditioned stimulus elicits as a result of the conditioning (training) procedure. At the start, the conditioned stimuluselicits no significant response. After conditioning, it elicits a conditioned response(Figure 10-2).

10.2.1.1 More examples of classical conditioning

You hear the sound of a dentist's drill shortly before the unpleasant experience of the drill on your teeth. From then on, the sound of a dentist's drillarouses anxiety.

Unconditioned stimulus = drilling → unconditioned response = tension

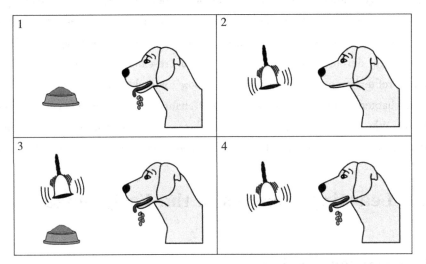

Figure 10-2 Classical conditioning

Conditioned stimulus = sound of the drill → conditioned response = tension

A nursing mother responds to her baby's cries by putting the baby to her breast, stimulating the flow of milk. After a few days of repetitions, the sound of the baby's cry is enough to start the milk flowing.

Unconditioned stimulus = baby sucking → unconditioned response = milk flow

Conditioned stimulus = baby's cry → conditioned response = milk flow

10.2.1.2 Additional phenomena of classical conditioning

The process that establishes or strengthens a conditioned response is known as acquisition. After discovering classical conditioning, Pavlov and others varied the procedures to produce other outcomes. Here are some of the main phenomena.

(1) Extinction

Suppose someone sounds a buzzer and then blows a puff of air into your eyes. After a few repetitions, you start to close your eyes as soon as you hear the buzzer. Now the buzzer sounds repeatedly without the puff of air. What do you do?

You blink your eyes the first time and perhaps the second and third times, but before long, you stop. This decrease of the conditioned response is called extinction. To extinguish a classically conditioned response, repeatedly present the conditioned stimulus (CS) without the unconditioned stimulus (UCS). That is, acquisition of a conditioned response (CR) occurs when the CS predicts the UCS, and extinction occurs when the CS no longer predicts the UCS.

Extinction is not the same as forgetting. Both weaken a learned response, but they arise in different ways. You forget during a long period without reminders or practice. Extinction occurs because of a specific experience—perceiving the conditioned stimulus without the unconditioned stimulus. If acquisition is learning to make a response, extinction is learning to inhibit it.

Don't be misled by connotations of the term extinction. After extinction of an animal or plant species, it is gone forever. In classical conditioning, extinction does not mean obliteration. Extinction suppresses a response. Think of it like extinguishing a fire: pouring water on a huge fire puts out the blazes, but a few smoldering embers may linger long afterward, and they might easily reignite the fire.

（2）Spontaneous recovery

Suppose you are in a classical-conditioning experiment. At first, you repeatedly hear a buzzer（CS）that precedes a puff of air to your eyes（UCS）. Then the buzzer stops predicting an air puff. After a few trials, your response to the buzzer extinguishes. Next you wait a while with nothing happening until suddenly you hear the buzzer again. What will you do? Chances are, you blink your eyes at least slightly. Spontaneous recovery is a temporary return of an extinguished response after a delay.

Why does spontaneous recovery occur? Think of it this way: at first, the buzzer predicted a puff of air to your eyes, and then it didn't. You behaved in accordance with the more recent experiences. Hours later, neither experience is much more recent than the other, nor are the effects of acquisition and extinction about equally strong.

10.2.2   Operant conditioning

Suppose a family in another country adopted you at birth. You then lived in a land with different language, customs, food, religion, and so forth. Undoubtedly you would be different in many ways. But would that alternative "you" have anything in common with the current "you"? Or does your culture and environment mold your behavior completely? The most extreme statement of environmental determinism came from John B. Watson, one of the founders of behaviorism, who said, give me a dozen healthy infants, well-formed, and my own specified world to bring them up in and I'll guarantee to take any one at random and train him to become any type of specialist I might select—doctor, lawyer, artist, merchant-chief, and yes, even beggar-man, thief, regardless of his talents, penchants, tendencies, abilities, vocations, and race of his ancestors.

Needless to say, Watson never had a chance to demonstrate his point. No one gave him a child and his own specified world. If he or anyone else really did have complete control of the environment, would it be possible to control a child's eventual fate? We may never know, ethics being what they are, after all. Still, one of the goals of researchers studying learning is to see what kinds of behavior change result from changes in the environment.

Operant behavior acts on the environment to produce reinforcement, and becomes strengthened by reinforcement.

e. g. , Skinner: experiment involving rat, a box and food.

One problem confronting any behavior researcher is how to define a response. Imagine watching children and trying to count "aggressive behaviors". What is an aggressive act and what isn't? Skinner simplified the measurement by simplifying the situation（Zuriff, 1995）: he set up a box, called an operant-conditioning chamber（or Skinner box）, in which a rat presses a lever or a pigeon pecks an illuminated "key" to receive food. He operationally defined the response as anything that the animal did to depress the lever or key. So if the rat pressed the lever with its snout instead of its paw, the response still counted. If the pigeon batted the key with its wing instead of pecking it with its beak, it still counted. The behavior was defined by its outcome, not by muscle movements（Figure 10-3）.

A pleasant consequence increases the chances of behavior to be repeated. An unpleasant consequences decreases the chances of behavior to be repeated. It is method used in a form of treatment called behavioral modification（Table 10-1）.

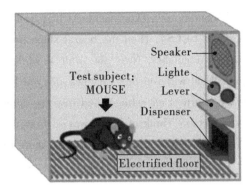

Figure 10-3   Skinner box

Table 10-1   The explanation of Skinner box

Items	Something given to the mouse	Something taken from the mouse
Increases Likelihood of repeated behavior	**Positive reinforcement** Mouse given food when lever pressed (after green light)	**Negative reinforcement** Loud noise stopped when lever pressed
Decreases Likelihood of repeated behavior	**Positive punishment** Mouse is shocked when lever pressed (after red light)	**Negative punishment** Not applicable in this scenario

10.2.2.1   Reinforcement and punishment

Some events work extremely well as reinforcers for some individuals and not others. Consider how many hours some people will play a video game just for a high score. In one quirky experiment, mother rats could press a lever to deliver extra baby rats into their cage. They kept on pressing and pressing, adding more and more babies. Is there any pattern as to what is a good reinforcer and what isn't?

We might guess that reinforcers are biologically useful to the individual, but many are not. For example, saccharin, a sweet but biologically useless chemical, can be a reinforcer. For many people, alcohol and tobacco are stronger reinforcers than vitamin-rich vegetables. So biological usefulness doesn't define reinforcement.

A useful way of defining reinforcement relies on the concept of equilibrium. If you could spend your day any way you wanted, how would you divide your time, on average? Let's suppose you might spend 30% of your day sleeping, 10% eating, 8% exercising, 11% reading, 9% talking with friends, 2% grooming, 2% playing the piano, and so forth. Now suppose something kept you away from one of these activities for a day or two. An opportunity to do that activity would get you back toward equilibrium. According to the disequilibrium principle of reinforcement, anything that prevents an activity produces disequilibrium, and an opportunity to return to equilibrium is reinforcing.

Of course, some activities are more insistent than others. If you have been deprived of oxygen, the opportunity to breathe is extremely reinforcing. If you have been deprived of reading time or telephone time, the reinforcement value is less.

10. 2. 2. 2   Primary and secondary reinforcers

Psychologists distinguish between primary reinforcers (or unconditioned reinforcers) that are reinforcing because of their own properties, and secondary reinforcers (or conditioned reinforcers) that became reinforcing by association with something else. Food and water are primary reinforcers. Money (a secondary reinforcer) becomes reinforcing because we can exchange it for food or other primary reinforcers. A student learns that a good grade wins approval, and an employee learns that increased productivity wins the employer's praise. We spend most of our time working for secondary reinforcers.

10. 2. 2. 3   Punishment

In contrast to a reinforcer, a punishment decreases the probability of a response. A reinforcer can be either a presentation of something (e. g. , receiving food) or a removal (e. g. , stopping pain). Similarly, punishment can be either a presentation of something (e. g. , receiving pain) or a removal (e. g. , withholding food). Punishment is most effective when it is quick and predictable. An uncertain or delayed punishment is less effective. For example, the burn you feel from touching a hot stove is highly effective in teaching you something to avoid. The threat that smoking cigarettes might give you cancer many years from now may also be effective, but less so. Punishments are not always effective. If the threat of punishment were always effective, the crime rate would be zero.

B. F. Skinner tested punishment in a famous laboratory study. He first trained food deprived rats to press a bar to get food and then he stopped reinforcing their presses. For the first 10 minutes, some rats not only failed to get food, but also received a slap on their paws every time they pressed the bar. The punished rats temporarily suppressed their pressing, but in the long run, they pressed as many times as did the unpunished rats. Skinner concluded that punishment produces no long-term effects.

That conclusion, however, is an overstatement. A better conclusion would be that punishment does not greatly weaken a response when no other response is available. Skinner's food-deprived rats had no other way to seek food(if someone punished you for breathing, you would continue breathing nevertheless).

Still, alternatives to punishment are often more effective. How could we get drivers to obey school-zone speed limits? Warning them of fines is not very effective. Even stationing police officers in the area has limited success. A surprisingly effective procedure is to post a driver feedback sign that posts the speed limit and an announcement of " your speed" based on a radar sensor. Just getting individual feedback heightens a driver's awareness of the law and likelihood of obeying it.

Is physical punishment of children, such as spanking, a good or bad idea? Spanking is illegal in many countries, mostly in Europe. Many psychologists strongly discourage spanking, recommending that parents simply reason with the child or use nonphysical methods of discipline, such as time out or loss of television or other privileges. What evidence backs this recommendation? All the research presents correlations between physical punishment and behavioral problems. Children who are frequently spanked tend to be ill behaved. You should see the problem in interpreting this result: it might mean that spanking causes misbehavior or it might mean that it'll behaved children provoke their parents to spank them. It could also mean that spanking is more common for families in stressful conditions, families with much parental conflict, or families with other factors that might lead to misbehaviors. A better type of research compares children who were frequently spanked to children from similar backgrounds who were frequently subjected to nonphysical punishment, such as time out. That type of research shows no difference between those spanked and those given other types of punishment. So it appears that misbehavior leads to

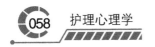

punishment (of whatever type) more than punishment leads to misbehavior.

The conclusions are different with regard to severe punishment bordering on child abuse. Likely outcomes then include antisocial behavior, low self-esteem, and hostility toward the parents, as well as increased risk for a lifetime of health problems.

Here is a summary table of the two kinds of conditionings(Table 10-2).

Table 10-2　Comparison of classical and operant conditioning

Subjects	Classical conditioning	Operant conditioning
Response	Involuntary, automatic	"Voluntary" operates on enviroment
Acquisition	Associating events; CS announces UCS	Associating response with a consequence (reinforcer or punisher)
Extinction	CR decreases when CS is repeatedly presented alone	Responding decreases when reinforcement stops
Cognitive processes	Subjects develop expectation that CS signals the arrival of UCS	Subjects develop expectation that a response will be reinforced or punished; they also exhibit latent learning, without reinforcement
Biological predispositions	Natural predispositions constrain what stimull and responses can easily be associated	Subjects best learn behaviors similar to their natural behaviors; unnatural behaviors instinctively drift back toward natural ones

10.2.3　Social learning theory

Social learning theory is based on the work of Alfred Bandura. It is also referred to as the social cognitive theory (SCT). The theory attempts to understand the process that is involved in explaining how we learn from each other. It focuses on learning that occurs by observing, imitating and modeling. It provides a framework for understanding, predicting and potentially changing human behavior.

Just as many birds learn their song from other birds, humans obviously learn much from each other. Just think of all the things you did not learn by trial and error. You don't throw on clothes at random and wait to see which clothes bring the best reinforcements. Instead, you copy the styles that other people are wearing. If you are cooking, you don't make up recipes at random. You start with what other people have recommended. If you are dancing, you don't randomly try every possible muscle movement. You copy what other people do.

According to the social-learning approach, we learn about many behaviors by observing the behaviors of others. For example, if you want to learn to drive a car, you start by watching people who are already skilled. When you try to drive, you receive reinforcement for driving well and punishments (possibly injuries!) If you drive badly, but your observations of others facilitate your progress.

Social learning is a type of operant conditioning, and the underlying mechanisms are similar. However, social information is usually quicker and more efficient than trying to learn something from scratch on your own. Behavior, personal factors and enviroment factors play important roles in the learning process. They are constantly influencing each other.

Bandura's doll: Albert Bandura studied the role of imitation for learning aggressive behavior. They asked two groups of children to watch films in which an adult or a cartoon character violently attacked an inflated "bobo" doll. Another group watched a different film. They then left the children in a room with a "bobo" doll. Only the children who had watched films with attacks on the doll attacked the doll themselves, using many of the same movements they had just seen. The clear implication is that children copy the aggressive behavior they have seen in others.

Chapter 11　Intelligence

Objectives

1. Master the concept of intelligence.
2. Familiarize yourself with intelligence research tasks.
3. Understand the theories of intelligence.

Section 1　Overview of Intelligence

What is intelligence? Different scholars have different understandings about it. Piaget argued that the essence of intelligence is biological adaptation, a special capacity between assimilation and adaptation. Wexler defined intelligence as "an aggregated or comprehensive capacity of the individual to act purposefully, think rationally, and cope effectively with circumstances". So comprehensive, because human behavior is characterized by the whole; so aggregation is because it is made up of elements or abilities.

11.1.1　Intelligence theory

Edward Lee Thorndike (1874—1949) was an American psychologist who was elected president of the American Psychological Association in 1912 and a member of the National Academy of Sciences in 1917. Thorndike proposed the "three-factor theory of intelligence". He believed that there could be abstract intelligence (including mental ability, especially the ability to process language and mathematical symbols), concrete intelligence (a person's ability to process things), and social intelligence (the ability of people to interact with each other), and that these three factors were jointly acted on by heredity, environment, and education.

(1) Abstract inteligence, which includes mental abilities, especially the ability to process language and mathematical symbols. A person with abstract intelligence is able to see the relationship between symbols to solve problems, such as doctors, lawyers, and mathematicians.

(2) Concrete intelligence is a person's ability to deal with things. For example, mechanical engineers and trained industrial engineers workers have a great deal of mechanical intelligence.

(3) Social intelligence, that is, the ability to deal with interactions between people. For example, salesmen, diplomats and politicians should have a communicative intelligence.

11.1.2　Multiple intelligences theory

Howard Gardner is the world famous educational psychologist, the most famous achievement is "multiple intelligences theory", known as the father of "multiple intelligences theory".

Gardner believes that the theory of multiple intelligences is supported by eight kinds of intelligences that exist relatively independently in individuals and are related to specific cognitive and knowledge domains: linguistic intelligence, rhythmic intelligence, mathematical intelligence, spatial intelligence, kinesthetic intelligence, introspection intelligence, communication intelligence and natural observation intelligence.

According to the theory of multiple intelligences, intelligence is the ability that individuals use to solve real problems they encounter or to produce and create effective products under the value standard of certain social or cultural environment. It contains the following meanings:

11.1.2.1　Each individual has its own intelligence

According to Gardner's multiple intelligences theory, as an individual, each of us has eight relatively independent intelligences at the same time. However, the eight relatively independent intelligences in each person are not absolutely isolated and irrelevant in real life, but organically combined in different ways and to different degrees. It is the combination of these eight intelligences in different ways and to different degrees in each person that makes each person's intelligence unique.

11.1.2.2　Development direction and degree of individual intelligence are influenced and restricted by environment and education

According to the theory of multiple intelligences, the development of individual intelligence is greatly influenced and restricted by the environment including social environment, natural environment and educational conditions, and its development direction and degree are different due to different environmental and educational conditions. Although there are eight kinds of intelligence in people under all kinds of environment and education conditions, the development direction and degree of people's intelligence under different environment and education conditions are obviously different.

11.1.2.3　Intelligence emphasizes the ability of individuals to solve practical problems and produce and create effective products needed by society

According to Gardner's multiple intelligences theory, intelligence should emphasize two abilities, one is the ability to solve practical problems, the other is the ability to produce and create effective products that society needs. According to Gardner's analysis, the traditional intelligence theory is produced in the modern industrial society that attaches great importance to verbal intelligence and logic-mathematical intelligence. Intelligence is interpreted as a kind of integrated ability with language ability and mathematical logic ability as the core.

11.1.2.4　Multiple intelligences theory attaches importance to the multi-dimensional perspective of viewing intelligence problems

In Gardner's view, the recognition that intelligence is composed of multiple equally important abilities rather than one or two core abilities, and that various intelligences are expressed in multiple dimensions and relatively independently rather than in an integrated way, should be the essence of the theory of multiple intelligences.

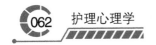

Section 2　Intelligence and IQ

IQ is the intelligence quotient. Intelligence is usually called wisdom, also known as intelligence. It is people's ability to understand objective things and use knowledge to solve practical problems. Intelligence includes many aspects, such as observation, memory, imagination, analysis and judgment ability, thinking ability, strain ability. The level of intelligence is usually expressed by the intelligence quotient, which is used to mark the level of intellectual development.

11.2.1　Intelligence test

Any of various tests of a person's general mental function. Also known as the general ability test. Intelligence tests are used to diagnose, collect basic data, assess mental disabilities, and assess treatment. Commonly used tests include the Binet – Simon Intelligence Scale, the Wexler Intelligence Scale, the Stanford–Binet Intelligence Scale, the Raven Standard Intelligence Test, the Army Group A Test, and the Army Group B Test.

In 1905, French psychologist Binet Alfred (1857—1911) and his students developed the world's first intelligence scale, according to which the average IQ of the average person is 100. In 1916, Professor Terman introduced this scale to the United States and revised it into the Stanford–Binet Intelligence Scale. The ratio of mental age and physical age was used as the index to assess the intelligence level of children. This ratio was called IQ, which was expressed by the formula: $IQ = MA(\text{mental age})/CA(\text{physical age}) \times 100$. In contemporary tests, the average level of performance for a given age is a score of 100. This intelligence is called proportional intelligence.

11.2.2　Other tests

(1) Aptitude test, also known as ability test, refers to the stable psychological characteristics of the test subjects, which are reflected in their cognitive ability. It mainly reflects the cognitive characteristics that are difficult to change under the influence of external environment, such as human observation, attention, memory, understanding, abstract thinking ability, judgment and reasoning ability, etc. This form is often used in the selection of business managers

(2) Achievement test, or achievement test, mainly examines the knowledge and skill level of the subject after learning and training. Because it is widely used in education, it is sometimes called educational test. According to different criteria, it can be classified more carefully. It is not only ability but also knowledge acquired through study that affects achievement test scores.

11.2.3　Because of factors affecting intelligence

11.2.3.1　Heredity

Genes related to IQ have been found to have different frequencydistributions in different ethnic groups, and ethnic groups with higher average IQ have more IQ genes than ethnic groups with lower average IQ. It is generally said that if the parents' IQ is high, the children's IQ will not be low. This genetic factor is also shown in the blood relationship, the parents of the same local, the average IQ of the children of

102；children born to parents who married in other provinces had IQ of 109. There was a marked increase in children with lower IQs if their parents were first cousins.

11.2.3.2　Mental disability

Down syndrome, autism, etc. For example, children with Down syndrome have obvious special features at birth and often present drowsiness and feeding difficulties, and their mental retardation gradually becomes obvious with age. Their IQ is 25 – 50, and motor and sexual development are delayed. The children have wide eye distance, low nose root, small eye cleft, oblique lateral eye, inner canthus fold, small outer ear, fat tongue, which often extends out of the mouth and salivates frequently. Short, head circumference is less than normal, head, back diameter short, occipital flatflat head, short neck, loose skin, bone age often lags behind the age, tooth delay and often dislocation, hair thin and soft and less, more in the middle, the anterior fontanelle closed late, top occipital middle line can have the third fontanelle, short limbs, due to ligament relaxation, joints can be excessively bent, fingers short, The middle gang bone dysplasia of the little finger causes the small finger to bend inward, the phalanx to be short, the palm trigeminal point to the distal end of the shift, common through the palm lines, straw shoes feet, about half of the children with the thumb ball are arch skin lines.

Children are often accompanied by congenital heart disease and other malformation, due to low immune function, prone to a variety of infections, the incidence of leukemia is 10–30 times higher than the general, such as survival to adult, often after 30 years old dementia symptoms.

11.2.3.3　Breast milk

Breast milk contains a variety of active substances to promote children's intellectual development, especially taurine which has an important impact on intellectual development is 10 times higher than milk. According to research, the IQ of children who grow up on breast milk is 3 – 10 points higher than that of children who grow up on milk substitute.

11.2.3.4　Diet

Monotonous diet leads to the deficiency of some trace elements, or too little diet, protein and other nutrients will lead to a serious lack of IQ development. High intake of heavy metals such as lead and copper can also affect IQ.

11.2.3.5　Weight

Weight of more than 20% of normal children, their vision, hearing, the ability to accept knowledge will be at a lower level. This is because obese children too much fat into the brain, will hinder the development of nerve cells and nerve fiber proliferation.

11.2.3.6　Environment

Living in a dull environment of children, such as abandoned babies, not maternal love and good education, IQ will be lower. According to the study, the average IQ of such children at the age of three was 60.5, where as the average IQ of children in good environment was 91.8.

11.2.3.7　Drugs

Some drugs will affect children's intelligence, such as long-term use of anti-epileptic drugs can make IQ low, when the drug stops for several years, IQ will be improved.

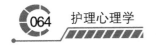

Section 3   Emotional Quotient

Emotional quotient(EQ), usually referred to as the emotional quotient, is a concept put forward by psychologists in recent years, which corresponds to IQ. Defined at a simple level, emotional intelligence is based on developing self-awareness and the ability to understand and express yourself.

According to Goleman and other researchers, emotional intelligence consists of five traits: self-awareness, control emotions, self-motivation, recognize others' emotions, and deal with interrelation.

(1)Self-awareness is to accurately identify and evaluate the emotions of oneself and others, to detect the changes of one's own emotions in time, and to summarize the causes of emotions.

(2) Control emotions is to adjust, guide, control and improve the emotions of oneself and others adaptively, which can make oneself get rid of strong anxiety and depression, cope with crisis actively, and enhance the emotional power to achieve goals. Self-control includes self-supervision, self-management, self-guidance, self-restraint and respect for reality. Respect for reality includes respect for your own reality, the reality of others and the reality of your surroundings.

(3)Self-motivation is to use emotional information, rectify emotions, enhance attention, mobilize their energy and vitality, establish goals adaptively, and achieve goals creatively. Self-encouragement is self-motivated, enterprising, enterprising, enterprising is to establish the goal of struggle, and actively work for it.

(4)Recognize others' emotions is the ability to consider others' emotional feelings and behavioral reasons, the ability and habit of empathy, the ability to understand and recognize emotional differences, the ability to live peacefully with people whose ideas are inconsistent with their own, the ability to understand others' feelings, the awareness of others' real needs, and empathy.

(5)Deal with interrelation is to be able to properly handle interpersonal issues and work harmoniously with others. Under the premise of increasingly detailed professional division of labor, mutual cooperation is becoming more and more important. The era calls for the spirit of teamwork, and the era requires mutual trust, mutual respect and mutual cooperation. The function of collaboration is to improve the performance of the organization, make the team work performance more than the simple sum of individual performance of the members, so as to form a strong team cohesion and overall combat effectiveness, and finally achieve the team goal. Only really into the team, to ensure the efficiency andquality of work.

Chapter 12   Motivation

Summary

Objectives
1. Master the concept of motivation.
2. Get familiar with types of motivation.
3. Understand the application of motivation in clinical nursing.

Section 1   General Concepts of Motivation

Motivation refers to the forces acting on or within ourselves to initiate, sustain and direct our behavior (Petri and Govern, 2004). It is an internal psychological process. It is a needs, desires, wants or drives within the individuals. It is the process of stimulating people to actions to accomplish the goals. Motivation can not be directly observed, but we can infer it indirectly through external manifestations such as the individual's choice of task, degree of effort, persistence in activities, and verbal expression.

12.1.1   Motivated behaviour

Motivation guides and activates behavior until the goal is achieved. Motivated behavioris goal directed. Motivated behavior varies from person to person, depending on the situation. The same motivation, different individuals can show different behavior; the same motivation, the same individual at different times can also show different behavior; the same behavior can be motivated by different reasons. Motivational behavior is influenced by many aspects, including internal and external needs. Motivation is the physical and psychological factors that cause us to act in a certain way at a certain time(Petri and Govern, 2004)。

12.1.2   A model of motivation

Many motivational activities begin with a need or an intrinsic lack or defect that leads to motivation (a state of energetic motivation) to achieve a desired goal, which, once achieved, creates a sense of satisfaction that feeds back into the original need or expectation (Figure 12-1). Motivation is the driven activation response (one or a series of actions) designed by an individual to achieve a goal (the goal of a motivational behavior).

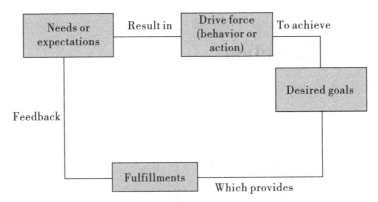

Figure 12-1 Basic model of motivation

Section 2　Types of Motives and Related Theories

12.2.1　Types of motives

Motives can be divided into three major categories: primary motives, stimulus motives, secondary motives.

12.2.1.1　Primary motives

The most important primary motives are hunger, thirst, avoidance of pain, air, sleep, excretion, and regulation of body temperature, and they are the ones that must be satisfied to sustain life. This is mainly about hunger.

Hunger is a physiological imbalance caused by the lack of food or nutrition in the body, which is manifested as a certain degree of nervousness, even some kind of torture and pain, thus forming the internal pressure of the individual, and drives the individual to produce eating activities. Hunger is related to many factors. First, hunger is associated with stomach contractions, but stomach contractions are not necessary to produce hunger, and many people who have had their stomachs removed can still feel hungry and eat as normal. Second, hunger is related to high and low blood sugar levels in the body. If blood sugar levels fall, hunger will increase. But insulin and blood sugar are not the only chemicals that regulate hunger. Moreover, the generation of hunger is also related to the function of some parts of the central nervous system. The so-called "hunger center" and "anorexia center" have been found in the hypothalamus of animals. The "hunger center" secretes a hunger-inducing hormone—orexin, and when mice are injected with this hormone, they turn into puffers. When the "anorexic center" is stimulated, the animal stops eating.

12.2.1.2　Stimulus motives

Stimulus motives includes activity, curiosity, exploration, manipulation (holding, touching) and contact (closeness, emotion), etc. It is the individual's need for stimulation and information or knowledge. These motivations drive people to actively explore the outside world. Note the introduction of interest here.

Interest is the psychological tendency of people to explore certain things or engage in certain activities. It is based on the needs of understanding or exploring the outside world, and it is an important motive to promote people to understand things and explore the truth. When an interest is directed toward an activity, this motivation is called a hobby. People will show great enthusiasm and attention to the things or activities that they are interested in. After the baby is born, it will react with surprise and excitement to the novel things in the environment, which is an individual inquiry into the environment.

12.2.1.3   Secondary motives

Many secondary motives are related to the learned need for power, subordination (the need to be with others), recognition, status, safety and achievement, which push individuals to actively interact with others, in the hope of gaining approval from society and others, and in the hope of participating in a certain social group and gaining a certain status within it. This is based on the need to learn, motivation and goals, such as money is worthless to a baby. It is through the process of learning that the paper becomes valuable and the motivation for action. This is mainly about the power motive.

Power motivation refers to the internal drive that people have to dominate and influence others and the surrounding environment. Under the control of power motive, people will actively participate and contribute in activities and have the desire to become leaders. From the point of individual behavior, power motive can be divided into individual power motive and social power motive. Individuals with individual power motive seek power to satisfy their personal desires or interests. Individuals with the motivation of social power seek rights for the sake of others. They show concern for society and others in their behaviors, and influence others with their personal knowledge and ideas.

12.2.2   Humanistic theory

The representative figures of humanistic theory are Abraham Maslow and Carl Rogers. Humanistic psychology believes that human nature is good, kind, people have free will, there is a need for self-realization.

12.2.2.1   Maslow's hierarchy of needs

Maslow put forward the hierarchy of needs theory (Figure 12 - 2). He believed that human needs are composed of five levels.

(1) Physiological needs

People's needs for food, water, air, excretion, sleep, sex, etc. They are the most important and powerful of all human needs.

(2) Safety needs

People's need for stability, security, protection, order, freedom from fear, anxiety and chaos. Safety needs arise if physiological needs are satisfied relatively adequately.

(3) Belongingness and love needs

The need to connect with other people, such as making friends, pursuing love, joining a group and achieving a status within it. If physiological needs and safety needs are met. The need to satisfy belonging and love arises.

(4) Esteem needs

The need for respect includes self-respect and the desire to be respected by others. The satisfaction of self-esteem needs will make individuals believe in their own value and make them more capable and creative. On the contrary, individuals with low self-esteem experience low self-esteem and lack confidence.

(5) Self-actualization needs

The need for self-actualization is manifested in people's pursuit of the maximum development of their ability or potential. The path to self-actualization variesfrom person to person. The need of self-actualization is the highest level of need, and its generation depends on the satisfaction of the aforementioned four needs.

Maslow believes that these five needs are all basic human needs. They are born with different levels, which motivate and guide individual behaviors. The lower the level of needs, the stronger the power will be, while the higher the level, the weaker the power will be. Only when the lower level needs are satisfied or partially satisfied can the higher level needs arise. Of course, there are exceptions to this rule. Some people are willing to sacrifice their lower needs in order to meet their higher needs. For example, some people are willing to sacrifice their lives for the realization of their beliefs and ideals.

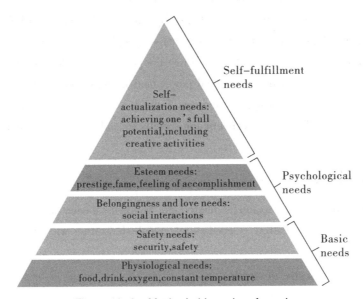

Figure 12-2　Maslow's hierarchy of needs

12.2.2.2 Types of motivation according to Maslow

Maslow divides motivation into two types: intrinsic motivation and extrinsic motivation.

(1) Intrinsic motivation

Motivation comes from the intrinsic drive, which is the motivation stimulated by the internal needs of individuals. What individuals do is based on their personal interests, challenges and enjoyment.

(2) Extrinsic motivation

Motivation comes from external driving factors, which is the behavioral motivation produced by individuals under the action of external requirements and external forces. What individuals do comes from factors other than people, such as rewards and tangible benefits.

Section 3   Application in Clinical Nursing

12.3.1   Application of needs in clinical nursing

In the clinical nursing work, patients because of the disease, the severity of the disease, education level, occupation, economic conditions and personality characteristics of different, in the clinical manifestations of the need to show characteristics are also different. Nurses should understand the necessity of meeting basic needs, as far as possible to meet the reasonable needs of patients, such as the patient's need for appropriate food, water or liquid, air or oxygen, understand the patient's pursuit of life safety, health and safety when the various psychological feelings, so as to carry out targeted nursing.

Nurses themselves should also have reasonable needs, and strive to pursue the need to meet, at the same time in the work of the pursuit of the needs of patients to meet, in order to achieve self-realization.

12.3.2   Application of motivation in clinical nursing

The motivation of seeking medical treatment and following medical advice of patients are closely related to the nursing work of nurses and affect the effect of nursing behavior. The nurse must remember that motivation plays a role in the daily relationship between patients, colleagues and herself. Understanding the patient's own motivations will help the nurse build a collaborative relationship between the patient and the healthcare team. Nurses should pay close attention to the motivation of patients, identify the possible motivation conflicts of patients, intentionally guide patients to realistic motivation in nursing work, actively cooperate with doctors and nurses in the treatment, and recover as soon as possible.

As an independent individual, nurses also have the motivation of pursuing achievement, right and communication, etc. At the same time, they should also be aware of the significance of nursing in the rehabilitation process of patients, and organically combine the two to achieve positive nursing effects.

Chapter 13　Emotion

Summary

> **Objectives**
> 1. Master the concept of emotion.
> 2. Familiar with emotional development.
> 3. Understand the elements of emotion.

Section 1　Concept and Elements of Emotion

13.1.1　Concept of emotion

Emotions refer to the experience of strong instinctive feelings usually directed toward a specific object and typically accompanied by physiological and behavioral changes in the body. Instinctive means automatic and does not require conscious thought. Emotion is a kind of psychological activity mediated by subjective desire and need. When the objective things or situations conform to the desires and needs of individuals, positive and positive emotions will be aroused. On the contrary, when the objective things or situations do not conform to the desires and needs of individuals, negative and negative emotions will be aroused. For example, patients who have been ill for a long time will feel happy if they can move freely after rehabilitation training, but they will be disappointed if they do not get good results from long – term exercise. Sometimes objective things or situations may satisfy one need of an individual, but not another, or even contradict other needs. Therefore, many things may cause very complex emotions, such as mixed feelings, tears and laughter, pain and happiness.

13.1.2　Elements of emotion

Emotion is a mixed psychological phenomenon, which consists of four elements: perception of stimuli, unique subjective experience, physiological arousal, and emotional expression.

13.1.2.1　Perception of stimuli

The perception of stimuli should first be aware of the existence of stimuli, so that stimuli can have an impact on individuals. Stimuli can be external natural or social situations, or internal physical or psychological feelings.

13.1.2.2　Subjective experience

Subjective experience is how individuals feel about different emotional states. Each emotion has different subjective experiences, which represent different feelings of people, such as happiness and sadness, and constitute the psychological content of emotions. Emotional experience is a kind of complex subjective feeling, and sometimes it is difficult to determine what objective stimulus is causing emotional experience. Moreover, different individuals may also have different emotions to the same stimulus, even if the same individual will make different emotional responses to the same stimulus at different times and under different conditions. For example, individuals may see the sunset as "the most beautiful sunset" when they are happy, and "the sunset is infinitely good but near dusk" when they are sad.

13.1.2.3 Physiological arousal

Physiological arousal refers to the physiological response produced by emotions, which involves a wide range of neural structures, such as the brain stem of the central nervous system, central gray matter, hypothalamus. Different emotions on physiological arousal level is different, such as happy, heart rhythm is normal, when rage when the heart speeds up, blood pressure increases, breathing rate increases, appear even intermittent or pause, vascular volume to reduce the pain, fear of the stomach will suspend activities, digestive juices also stopped secretion, sweat gland secretion changes. People can feel themselves in emotional state, but they can not control their emotions well, because the autonomic nervous system controlling emotions is generally not controlled by personal will.

13.1.2.4 Emotional expression

It is a quantified form of movement of various parts of the body during the occurrence of emotional states, including facial expression, posture expression and intonation expression. A facial expression is a pattern of changes in all facial muscles. Such as happy forehead brow flat, cheek, mouth turned up. Facial expressions are pan – cultural. The same facial expression will be recognized and used by people from different cultural backgrounds to express the same emotional experience. Facial expression recognition research has also found that the most recognizable expressions are happiness and pain, the less recognizable are fear and sadness, and the least recognizable are doubt and pity. In general, the more complex the emotional component, the harder the expression is to recognize. Posture expression refers to the expression and movement of other parts of the body other than the face. For example, dancing when happy, beating their chests when sad, being cocky when successful, dejected when failed. Posture expression are not cross-cultural and are influenced by different cultures. Intonation expression refers to the expression of emotion in the pitch, rhythm and speed of speech. Such as excited voice high sharp, happy intonation excited, fast, painful intonation low, slow rhythm, nervous incoherent, tone has a sudden change, often interrupted speech and slip of the tongue.

Section 2 Emotional Development and Influencing Factors

13.2.1 Emotional development

As a child grows and develops his motor skills, he also develops his emotions, which constantly diverge and diversify. Emotional changes develop faster before the age of 2. At 4–6 weeks, children show social smiles in the face of smiles. At 3–4 months, he gets upset when you're angry and curious when he hears loud noises. At 5–7 months of age, people are afraid of strangers and frightened by loud noises. At 6–

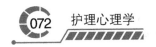

8 months, you have shyness, you have a sense of shame, you have an aversion to things. At 24 months, emotions are more intense and you learn to regulate your emotions.

13.2.2 Factors that affect emotional development

Although diffuse emotions may appear soon after birth, emotional development is a result of maturity and learning. Factors that influence emotional development include genetics, neurological (brain), cognitive – psychological processes, coping and cultural factors, environmental conditions, daily life experiences, and personal health. The interplay of these factors makes us unique.

One of the genetic factors that influence mood development is temperament. Temperament broadly refers to the individual differences in biological behavior, is a stable psychological characteristics in the intensity, speed, flexibility and directivity of psychological activities, that is, we usually say disposition, nature. The person's temperament difference is formed a priori, subject to the characteristic restriction of nervous system activity process, will never change, it just develops as time. Such as children just a birth, some children love to cry active, some children smooth quiet, this first show the difference is temperament difference. These temperamental differences also affect how babies relate to their parents, who encourage quiet, reserved children more than active ones.

Temperament is human nature, there is no good or bad. He only paints a certain color to people's words and deeds, but he can not determine people's social value, nor directly has the meaning of social moral evaluation. A person's lively and steady can not determine his way of doing things. People of any temperament type can be virtuous and beneficial to society, or they can be corrupt and harmful to society. Temperament affects people's choice of career, but can not determine a person's achievement, any temperament, as long as through their own efforts, can make achievements in different fields of practice, but may also become a mediocre person.

Modern temperament theory divides temperament into four typical types: choleric, sanguine, mucous, and depressive. Choleric type of people have low sensitivity, high tolerance, strong emotional experience, rapid outbreak, rapid calm, flexible but careless thinking, energetic, aggressive, brave and decisive, enthusiastic and straightforward, quick action; but they are often thoughtless, rash, emotional and self – willed. Sanguine type of people emotional rich, exposed, but unstable, quick thinking, but not to understand, lively and active, good at communication, strong adaptability; this type of person lacks patience and perseverance, has poor stability, and changes his mind. People of this type of mucus have smooth emotions, plain expression, thoughtful and meticulous thinking, quiet and calm, and strong self–control; but this type of people lack vitality, thinking flexibility is slightly poor, slow action, poor initiative. Depressive type of person has profound emotional experience, delicate and lasting, emotional depression, sentimentality, keen thinking, rich imagination, strong self–control, but this type of person is slow, soft and timid, indecisive. In real life, the person of single temperament is not much, most of the people are the mixture of four kinds of temperament.

Individual differences between people, some babies happy, cheerful, eat sleep pattern, adapt to the new environment quickly; others may warm up slowly, aloof, emotional, need longer time to adapt to the new environment. Some babies picky, fear, more intense reaction, which requires the nurse can timely understand the reaction of the patients in the clinical work, understand the attachment relationship between children and parents or other caregivers, sensitively and specifically treat different children, and better care for them.

Chapter 14   Memory

Summary

Objectives
1. Master the concept of memory.
2. Familiar with the process of forgetting.
3. Understand the types of memory.

Section 1   Concept and Types of Memory

14.1.1   Concept of memory

Memory processes information similar to a computer in that a file is written, stored on a specific disk drive, and then retrieved from the drive when needed. The things people have felt, the problems they have thought, the emotions they have experienced or the activities they have engaged in will leave different degrees of impressions in their minds. Some of these impressions become experience, which can be retained for a long time and can be recovered under certain conditions. This is memory.

In the term of information processing, memory is the process by which the human brain encodes, stores and extracts information from the outside world. Encoding is the mental representation of information in order to keep it in our memory (place it in memory). This is the initial stage of memory, the process of acquiring individual experience, equivalent to the "memorization" stage in memory. In the process of memory, there are different levels or levels of encoding, mainly visual, auditory and semantic encoding, and different encoding methods have different effects on memory.

Storage is the process of putting encoded information into relatively permanent storage that can be recalled later (held in memory). It is the intermediate link of information encoding and extraction and plays an important role in the process of memory. Storage is an active process, and the information stored is not static, changing both in content and quantity. In terms of quantity, the amount of stored information gradually decreases with the passage of time; in terms of content, the stored content becomes more brief and general, more complete, reasonable and meaningful, more specific or more exaggerated and prominent, and the unimportant details will gradually tend to disappear.

Retrieval is the process of obtaining or recalling information from short – or long – term storage (recovery from memory). Is the last stage of the memory process, equivalent to the "recall" stage of memory. There are two basic forms of recall and recognition. Experienced things are not in front of the

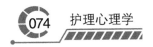

eyes,can recall it back to the process,called recall. The process of recognizing an experienced object when it appears again is called recognition. For example,in the exam,filling in the blanks is the process of recall,multiple choice is the process of recognition.

The three basic processes of memory are closely linked. In general,if the encoding is better and the storage is better,the extraction is easier.

14.1.2 Types of memory

According to the length of information retention time,memory is divided into sensory memory,short-term memory and long-term memory.

14.1.2.1 Sensory memory

When objective stimuli stop acting,sensory information is preserved in a very short period of time. This kind of memory is called sensory memory or sensory registration. Sensory memory is the process in which an individual receives information from the environment,which is the beginning stage of the memory system. The storage time of information in the brain is very short, ranging from 0.25 to 4.00 s. Sensory memory has a large capacity,but only the information that can attract the attention of the individual and be recognized in time has a chance to enter the short-term memory,and the information that is not noticed quickly disappears. Although the information is held in sensory memory for a short time,it can be very useful. When watching movies and television,the timing of eye movements and blinks does not affect the coherence of our perception due to sensory memory.

14.1.2.2 Short-term memory

Short-term memory refers to the ability to hold a limited amount of information for a short period of time,ranging from 5 seconds to 1 minutes. It is an intermediatestage between sensory and long-term memory and has a limited capacity of 7±2 blocks. There are many factors that affect the effect of short-term memory encoding. Arousal state is the excitability level of the cerebral cortex,which directly affects the effect of memory encoding. Studies have shown that memory span peaks around 10:30 a.m. ,declines throughout the afternoon,and is least productive in the evening. Processing depth is also a factor affecting short-term memory encoding. Finally,chunking or enlarging the amount of information contained in each block can improve the encoding of memory. For example,look up a phone number and dial it quickly before forgetting it. If you repeat it over and over again,you'll be able to keep it in short-term memory longer. If you're more involved,such as taking notes and reviewing as well as listening to a lecture,the information will be encoded into long-term memory.

14.1.2.3 Long-term memory

Long-term memory is a memory that lasts longer than 1 minutes,up to many years,or even a lifetime. There is no limit to capacity; the source of information is mostly the processing of short-term memory content,and some of the information is obtained at once because of the deep impression. Long-term memory stores all our past experience and knowledge,linking the past and present of people's mental activities,is the basic function of our study,work and life. The state of mind at the time of encoding affects the encoding of long-term memories,and studies have found that intentional encoding is better than automatic encoding. The depth of processing also affects the encoding of long-term memories. The extraction of information from long-term memory depends on the way the information is stored and the amount of interference from related information. In information storage,accuracy can vary and sometimes distort.

Sensory, short – term, and long – term memory are not either – or types of memory. The difference between them is not only the length of information retention time or the amount of information retention, but they are in different stages from their information processing in the memory system, and there is a continuous interaction between them. As shown in Figure 14 – 1, information acts on the senses and generates sensory memory. The impressive or processed information in the sensory memory goes into the short–term memory, while other information disappears. The information entered into short – term memory becomes long – term memory after repeated processing. The unprocessed information disappears, and the information in long–term memory can also be extracted into short–term memory.

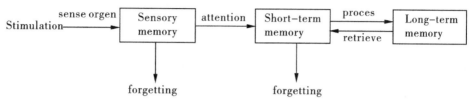

Figure 14-1   Tertiary processing model of memory

Section 2   Forgetting

Forgetting refers to inability to retrieve, recall or recognize information that was stored or is still stored in the long term memory.

14.2.1   Process of forgetting

The first person to study forgetting was the German psychologist Thomas Ebbinghaus. Using meaningless syllables as memorizing materials, he asked the subjects to repeat learning, measured the amount of memory retention by saving method, and plotted the experimental results into a curve, which was known as the Ebbinghaus forgetting curve (Figure 14–2). As can be seen from the figure, forgetting begins immediately after learning, and the process of forgetting progresses rapidly at first and gradually slows down thereafter.

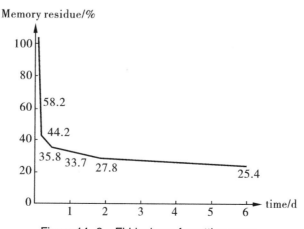

Figure 14-2   Ebbinghaus forgetting curve

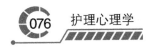

14.2.2　Cause of forgetting

According to the interference theory, forgetting is the inability to recall specific information due to memory blockage caused by other related memories. For example, if you have to take several tests on the same day, you may get confused and forgotten about what you have prepared for them. Proactive inhibition and retroactive inhibition are good proof of interference theory.

Proactive inhibition is the interference of the learned material on the learned material after memorizing and recalling. Retroactive inhibition is the interference effect of later learning material on memory and recall of the first learning material. For example, when reciting a poem, the first half and the second half of the poem are generally remembered quickly and firmly, while the middle part is recognized slowly and forgotten quickly, because the middle part is affected by the dual effects of proactive inhibition and retroactive inhibition. This also reminds us to pay attention to the sequence position of the materials when learning, to study the order of the learning materials, the middle part should also be more review and consolidation, in case of forgetting.

Amnesia is a temporary or permanent loss of memory after a blow or injury to the brain, which can be caused by disease or trauma.

Chapter 15   Personality

Summary

Objectives
1. Outline the 3 theories to personality development.
2. Identify the factors influence personality.
3. Define personality, the purpose of studying personality.

Section 1   Definition and Significance of Personality

15.1.1   Definition

Personality is the characteristics pattern of thinking, feeling and behaving of an individual. It is believed that personality arises from within the individual and remains fairly consistent throughout life.

What is human nature? The seventeenth-century philosopher Thomas Hobbes argued that humans are by nature selfish. Life in a state of nature, he said, is "nasty, brutish, and short." The eighteenth-century political philosopher Jean-Jacques Rousseau disagreed, maintaining that people are naturally good. Rational people acting freely, he maintained, would advance the welfare of all.

The debate between those two viewpoints survives in theories of personality. Sigmund Freud held that people are born with impulses that must be held in check if civilization is to survive. Carl Rogers believed that people seek good and noble goals after they have been freed from unnecessary restraints.

Which point of view is correct? Way down deep, are we good, bad, both, or neither? What is the basic nature of human personality?

The term personality comes from the Latin word "persona", meaning "mask". In the plays of ancient Greece and Rome, actors wore masks to indicate their characters. Unlike a mask, however, the term personality implies something stable. Personality consists of all the consistent ways in which the behavior of one person differs from that of others, especially in social situations(differences in learning, memory, sensation, or athletic skills are generally not considered personality).

15.1.2   Purpose of studying personality

(1)Important guidelines regarding how best to understand an individual patient's illness.

(2)How best to care for each patient as an individual.

(3)Provide insight into how nurse approaches his or her role in caring for the patient.

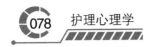

Section 2　Development of Personality

15.2.1　Three aspects of personality according to behavierist

(1) Extroversion/Introversion (E)

Extraverts are sociable and crave excitement and change, and thus can become bored easily. They are more likely to take risks and be thrill seekers. Eysenck argues that this is because they inherit an under aroused nervous system and so seek stimulation to restore the level of optimum stimulation. Introverts on the other hand lie at the other end of this scale, being quiet and reserved. They are already over-aroused and shut sensation and stimulation. Introverts are reserved, plan their actions and control their emotions. They tend to be serious, reliable and pessimistic.

(2) Neuroticism/Stability (N)

A person's level of neuroticism is determined by the reactivity of their sympathetic nervous system. A stable person's nervous system will generally be less reactive to stressful situations, remaining calm and levelheaded. Someone high in neuroticism on the other hand will be much more unstable, and prone to overreacting to stimuli and may be quick to worry, anger or fear. They are overly emotional and find it difficult to calm down once upset.

(3) Psychoticism/Normality

Eysenck later added a third trait / dimension—psychoticism, e. g. , lacking in empathy, cruel, a loner, aggressive and troublesome. This has been related to high levels of testosterone. The higher the testosterone, the higher the level of psychoticism, with low levels related to more normal balanced behavior.

15.2.2　Psychoanalytic approach

Personality development depends on the interaction of instinct (nature) and environment (parental influence) during the first 5 years of life. Environmental and parental experiences during childhood influence an individual's personality during adulthood. For example, during the first 2 years of life, the infant who is neglected (insufficiently fed) or who is over-protected (over-fed) might become an orally fixated person.

15.2.2.1　Sigmund Freud's psychosexual stages

(1) The oral stage

In the oral stage, from birth to about age 1, the infant derives intense pleasure from stimulation of the mouth, particularly while sucking at the mother's breast. According to Freud, someone fixated at this stage continues to receive great pleasure from eating, drinking, and smoking and may also have lasting concerns with dependence and independence.

(2) The anal stage

At about age 2, children enter the anal stage, when they get psychosexual pleasure from the sensations of bowel movements. if toilet training is too strict—or too lenient—the child becomes fixated at this stage. someone fixated at the anal stage goes through life "holding things back"—being orderly, stingy, and stubborn—or less commonly, goes to the opposite extreme, becoming messy andwasteful.

（3）The phallic stage

Beginning at age 3, in the phallic stage, children begin to play with their genitals and according to Freud become sexually attracted to the opposite – sex parent. Freud claimed that every boy is afraid of having his penis cut off, whereas girls develop "penis envy. "These ideas have always been doubtful, and they have few defenders today.

（4）The latent period

From about age 5 or 6 until adolescence, Freud said, most children enter a latent period in which they suppress their psychosexual interest. At this time, they play mostly with peers of their own sex. The latent period is evidently a product of European culture and does not appear in all societies.

（5）The genital stage

Beginning at puberty, young people take a strong sexual interest in other people. This is known as the genital stage. According to Freud, anyone who has fixated a great deal of libido in an earlier stage has little libido left for the genital stage. But people who have successfully negotiated the earlier stages now derive primary satisfaction from sexual intercourse（Table 15-1）.

Table 15-1　Sigmund Freud's psychosexual stages

Stage	Age range	What happens at this stage?
Oral stage	0-1 year old	Children derive pleasure from oral activities, including sucking and tasting. They like to put things in their mouth
Anal stage	2-3 years old	Children begin potty training
Phallic stage	3-6 years old	Boys are more attached to their mother, while girls are more attached to their father
Latency stage	6 years old to puberty	Children spend more time and interact mostly with same sex peers
Genital stage	Beyond puberty	Individuals are attracted to opposite sex peers

15.2.2.2　Structure of personality

According to Freud, our personality develops from a conflict between two forces: our biological aggressive and pleasure – seeking drives versus our internal (socialized) control over these drives. Our personality is the result of our efforts to balance these two competing forces. Freud suggested that we can understand this by imagining three interacting systems within our minds. He called them the id, ego, and superego. According to Freud, our personality develops from a conflict between two forces: id and superego. Our personality (ego) is the result of our efforts to balance these two competing forces.

15.2.2.3　Defense mechanism

（1）Repression

The defense mechanism of repression is motivated removal of something to the unconscious—rejecting unacceptable thoughts, desires, and memories. For example, someone who has an unacceptable sexual impulse might become unaware of it. Freud maintained that people repress painful, traumatic memories. repressed material is removed from consciousness but not forgotten. Freud once compared a repressed thought to a rowdy person expelled from a polite room who continues banging on the door, trying to get back in.

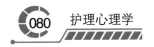

（2）Denial

The refusal to believe unpleasant information（"this can't be happening"）is denial. Whereas repression is the motivated removal of information from consciousness, denial is an assertion that the information is incorrect, generally accompanied by a wish-fulfilling fantasy. For example, someone with an alcohol problem may insist, "I'm not an alcoholic. I can take it or leave it." Someone whose marriage is headed for divorce may insist that all is going well. People who are about to get fired may believe that they are highly successful on the job.

（3）Rationalization

When people attempt to show that their actions are justifiable, they are using rationalization. For example, a student who wants to go to the movies says: "More studying won't do me any good anyway." Someone who takes unfair advantage of another says: "Learning to deal with disappointment will make him a better person."

（4）Displacement

By diverting a behavior or thought away from its natural target toward a less threatening target, displacement lets people engage in the behavior with less anxiety. For example, if you are angry with your employer or your professor, you might yell at someone else.

（5）Projection

Attributing one's own undesirable characteristics to other people is known as projection. If someone tells you to stop being angry, you might reply: "I'm not angry! you're the one who's angry!" suggesting that other people have your faults might make the faults seem less threatening. For example, someone who secretly enjoys pornography might accuse other people of enjoying it. However, the research finds that people using projection do not ordinarily decrease their anxiety or their awareness of their own faults.

（6）Reaction formation

To avoid awareness of some weakness, people sometimes use reaction formation to present themselves as the opposite of what they really are. In other words, they go to the opposite extreme. A man troubled by doubts about his religious faith might try to convert others to the faith. Someone with unacceptable aggressive tendencies might join a group dedicated to preventing violence.

（7）Sublimation

The transformation of sexual or aggressive energies into culturally acceptable, even admirable, behaviors is sublimation. according to Freud, sublimation lets someone express an impulse without admitting its existence. For example, painting and sculpture may represent a sublimation of sexual impulses. Someone may sublimate aggressive impulses by becoming a surgeon. Sublimation is the one proposed defense mechanism that is associated with socially constructive behavior. However, if the true motives of a painter are sexual and the true motives of a surgeon are violent, they are well hidden indeed.

15.2.3 Humanistic approach

Concerned with the individual's personal view of the world, his self-concept and his ability to reach his fullest potential. People are responsible for their lives and actions and have the freedom and will to change their attitudes and behavior.

Humanistic theories have their philosophical roots in phenomenology and existentialism, and some would say they're more "philosophical" than "psychological". They're concerned with characteristics that are distinctively and uniquely human, in particular experience, uniqueness, meaning, freedom and choice. We have first-hand experience of ourselves as people, and Rogers' theory in particular is centered around the self-concept.

What Rogers and Maslow have in common is their positive evaluation of human nature, a belief in the individual's potential for personal growth (self-actualization). But while Maslow's theory is commonly referred to as a " psychology of being " (self-actualization is an end in itself and lies at the peak of his hierarchy of needs), Rogers' is a " psychology of becoming " (it focuses on the process of becoming a " fully functioning person ").

According to Torrance and Jordan, Maslow's account of human needs emphasizes the central role for the biological sciences in nursing theory and practice. Nurses encounter individuals with ill health and disease on a daily basis and therefore clinical nursing practice is moulded around the individual's physiological and psychological responses to these health problems. Although nursing practice clearly has a role beyond illness (e. g. , health education and promotion), its main focus remains with people who are ill. Torrance and Jordan argue that, in the broader view, nursing aims to help with both deficit and growth needs, but it has to ensure that immediate physiological and safety needs are met. If the nurse/patient relationship is effective in meeting these basic needs, it can then offer assistance in meeting higher-level needs. However, it does appear that people become patients because illness interferes with their ability to meet the lower-level needs from their own resources.

Concept of self and experiences related to self is central to personality development. The direction of our movement basically is towards self-actualization. Rogers further divided the self into two categories: the ideal self and the real self. If there is incongruent, it will result in possible confusion, tension, and maladaptive behavior.

Chapter 16   Disease

Objectives

1. Master the factors affecting the disease and the psychological reactions of patients with malignant tumors.
2. Familiar with the classification of diseases, the performance of patient role adaptation difficulties, and the role of nurses.
3. Understand the basic concepts of the disease and the patient's role characteristics.

Section 1   Overview

16. 1. 1   Basic concepts

Health means that in the process of life activities, through the regulation of nerves and humors, the function, metabolism and morphological structure of various organs maintain a normal coordination relationship, and the body maintains a relative balance with the changing external environment.

When the World Health Organization was established in 1946, it clearly stated in the charter: "Health is not only the absence of disease and physical weakness, but a state of physical, psychological and social perfection." In 1990, health has a new definition, that is, "Health is not just the absence of disease, but includes physical health, mental health, social well-being and moral health."

Sickness refers to the subjective experience that an individual can feel sickor unwell, which often can not be directly verified, affects their physical and mental state, makes them feel uncomfortable or some kind of pain, and is accompanied by different degrees of physical, psychological, and social dysfunction, and is caused by this leads to medical seeking behavior. The feeling of illness may be due to physical reactions such as pain caused by a certain disease, or it may be affected by psychological, social and other factors, resulting in individual physical and psychological reactions.

Disease refers to that due to the invasion of pathogenic factors, the normal physiological and psychological activities deviate from the normal, the functional coordination and order of the body system are destroyed, and the social adaptability is damaged. In most diseases, the body responds to the damage caused by the cause in a series of anti – damage responses, and the result may be recovery of the disease or disability, or even death of the individual. The disturbance of homeostasis regulation, damage and anti – damage responses, are manifested in the abnormal changes of various complex functions, metabolism and morphological structures during the disease process, and these changes in turn can cause changes between the various organ systems of the body and between the body and the external environment. The coordination relationship of people is impaired, resulting in various symptoms, signs and behavioral abnormalities, especially the weakening or even loss of the ability to adapt to the environment and labor.

Illness and ailment are both different and related. Disease refers to the damage to the organs, tissues or psychology of the human body, symptoms, corresponding signs or behavioral characteristics, positive findings in laboratory tests, and a decline in the patient's social function. Sickness is a subjective experience. Individuals who have a feeling of illness may appear to seek medical treatment, but a feeling of illness is not necessarily a disease. However, some diseases are serious, but the patient does not feel sick, such as cancer found in routine physical examination.

Patients have a narrow sense and a broad sense. In a narrow sense, patients refer to people who suffer from various physical diseases, psychosomatic diseases or mental disorders. They are called patients regardless of whether they seek medical treatment or not. It also includes those who only have a sense of disease but have not found any physical pathological changes clinically. In a broad sense, patients refer to all objects receiving medical and health services, including healthy people.

16.1.2   Classification of diseases

According to the speed of onset and progression, diseases can be divided into acute diseases and chronic diseases.

Acute disease refers to a disease with abrupt onset, rapid disease progression and severe symptoms, such as acute appendicitis. According to its disease can be divided into mild, moderate and severe. Mild often refers to small local injuries or lesions that have little impact on the body; moderate often refers to lesions that have affected body functions or behaviors; severe refers to lesions that seriously affect body functions or behaviors. For mild patients, short-term treatment can be done at home, such as mild cough, a small amount of diarrhea, small skin abrasions; if it improves after treatment, there is no need to go to the hospital, if it does not improve or worsens after treatment, you should go to the hospital for treatment. For moderate and severe illness, seek medical attention as soon as possible or urgently.

Chronic disease is a gradual disease with less severe symptoms, with insidious onset, long course of disease and unhealed disease, long duration, 6 months or more, and complex etiology. Affect the patient's ability to work and quality of life, such as diabetes and heart disease.

16.1.3   The factor that affect the disease

16.1.3.1   Age

The occurrence of age-related diseases has a certain relationship with age. With the increase of age, the possibility of people getting sick is greater. Many studies have found that the incidence of Alzheimer's disease will gradually increase after the age of 65, and the seventies and eighties are more concentrated onset stages.

16.1.3.2   Gender

In some diseases, gender is different, the incidence is different. Studies have shown that women are twice as likely to suffer from depression as men. At the same time, different genders have different types

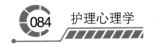

of cancer, such as breast cancer in women and prostate cancer in men.

16.1.3.3　Economic status

The economic status of individuals affects their material living standards to a certain extent. Poor economy can lead to less intake of protein, fat, vitamins, etc. , resulting in malnutrition. The economy is better, and excessive food intake can lead to excess weight, which affects health.

16.1.3.4　Social culture

Social culture is a general term for various cultural phenomena and cultural activities that are closely related to the production and life of the masses at the grassroots level, created by the grassroots people, have regional, ethnic or group characteristics, and exert extensive influence on social groups. Different countries and different ethnic groups have different social cultures, different social cultures have different views on the same disease, and different eras have different views on the unified disease.

16.1.3.5　Personality

Perfection of personality is an important symbol of health. Perfection of personality refers to a sound and unified personality, ability, personality, temperament, interest, world outlook and other aspects can be developed harmoniously and balanced, without obvious defects and deviations. Studies have found that people with type A behavior are prone to coronary heart disease, and people with type C behavior are prone to malignant tumors.

16.1.3.6　Lifestyle

According to statistics, unhealthy lifestyles such as smoking, alcoholism, drug abuse, overeating and obesity, and lack of exercise are important factors that affect human health.

16.1.3.7　Inherited

Genetic factors directly cause disease mainly through genetic mutations and chromosomal aberrations. Gene mutations cause molecular diseases, such as hemophilia, and chromosomal aberrations cause chromosomal diseases, which have reached hundreds of types, such as hermaphroditism caused by sex chromosome aberrations.

16.1.4　The stage of the disease

American scholar Suchman, observing the procedures of medical activities, divides the disease into five stages: symptom experience, assume on the role of the patient, access to medical services, dependent, healing and recovery.

16.1.4.1　Symptom experience

At this stage, the individual feels unwell, and often can not diagnose the problem by himself due to lack of medical knowledge. At this time, patients often have three symptoms, which are the physical experience of symptoms, cognitive aspects and emotional responses. At the end of this stage, it is often recognized that this is a symptom of a disease.

16.1.4.2　Assume the role of the patient

If symptoms persist, the individual will assume the role of the patient and seek support from family or others. He will then be freed from his normal duties and role expectations, and will no longer fulfill the obligations and responsibilities of his normal role. At this stage, the patient will have negative emotions, such as fear, anxiety, anger. Patients may experience delays in seeking medical attention.

16.1.4.3 Access to medical services

At this stage, patients will seek treatment on their own initiative or after being urged by others, and doctors will use professional knowledge to determine whether they are ill. If the patient receives a doctor's diagnosis, the patient will receive the treatment prescribed by the doctor. Patients typically ask about three types of information, whether it is a disease, an explanation of symptoms, and a prognosis. Some patients are sceptical about the doctor's diagnosis and refuse treatment.

16.1.4.4 Dependent

Patients are eager to recover as soon as possible, so they can actively receive treatment and care. Patients are eager to get help and care from the people around them, and they are psychologically and behaviorally dependent on doctors and nurses. Even some patients are too concerned about the disease and rely too much on the hospital environment. After the treatment improves or recovers, they are unwilling to change from the role of the patient to the normal role, and are unwilling to leave the medical staff.

16.1.4.5 Healing and recovery

At this stage, the symptoms of the disease disappear, and the patient begins to return to a healthy state. In general, the patient can return to the previous living state, but some diseases can lead to a long-term decline in the patient's social function.

16.1.5 The impact of the disease on patients, families and society

Illness is not an isolated life event that causes some changes in patients and their families. These changes vary depending on the type, severity and duration of the disease, cost of treatment, lifestyle changes, role changes and adjustments, etc.

16.1.5.1 The impact of the disease on the patient

(1) Influence of personal behavior and emotions

Generally speaking, the changes in individual behavior and emotions caused by the disease can vary according to the nature of the disease and the attitudes of the patient and others towards the disease. Usually, short-term, non-life-threatening illnesses do not cause many emotional and behavioral changes in patients, but severe illness, especially life - threatening illnesses, can cause strong behavioral and emotional changes, such as anxiety, shock, anger.

(2) Influence of personal autonomy and lifestyle

Diseases can usually reduce personal autonomy and lead to more clumps or medical compliance.

(3) Effects on body image

Some diseases can cause changes in the patient's body image, resulting in a series of psychological reactions in patients and their families. The magnitude of the response depends on the type of appearance change, the ability of the patient and family to adapt, the abruptness of the appearance change, and the health of the support system.

(4) Effects on self-concept

Self-concept is affected by many factors, such as loss of a certain part or function of the body, pain, dependence on others, lack of ability to participate in social activities.

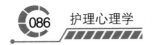

16.1.5.2　The impact of the disease on the family

（1）Economic impact

After an individual falls ill, he or she needs to go to the hospital for treatment or inpatient treatment, or even surgical treatment, which will increase family expenses and bring certain economic burdens to the family. In order to reduce the financial burden of the family, some patients will choose to give up treatment, and even have extreme behaviors, thus affecting the treatment and recovery of the disease. If the patient is the main source of the family's economic income, it will increase the family's economic burden and have a more serious impact on the family.

（2）Excessive psychological pressure on family members

The family members of patients not only have to assume the original family role of the patient, but also invest a lot of time and energy to take care of the patient, which increases the burden on family members and generates corresponding psychological pressure.

（3）Changes in family roles

The effect of illness on changes in family roles may be short or long, depending on the nature of the disease. Short-term illness has less impact on patient and family functioning.

16.1.5.3　The impact of disease on society

（1）Reducing social productivity

Everyone contributes to society with their social roles at work. After individual patients change their roles, they are temporarily or long-term exempt from social responsibilities and can not assume their original social roles. Social productivity will definitely be reduced.

（2）Consumption of social medical resources

Diagnosis and treatment of diseases will consume certain social medical resources.

（3）Cause infection and threaten the health of others

Certain infectious diseases, such as hepatitis, tuberculosis, will spread among the crowd, infect others, and affect the health of others if proper measures are not taken.

Section 2　Roles of Patiens and Nurses

16.2.1　Role of the patient

When a person is diagnosed with a disease, he acquires another role, the patient role, also known as patient status.

16.2.1.1　Characteristics of the patient's role

（1）Degradation of social role

After an individual becomes ill, he can be released from his original social role, his original social and family responsibilities, rights and obligations are exempted as appropriate, and he can get rest or receive medical treatment according to the nature and severity of the disease help.

（2）Decreased self-control ability

After illness, individuals will appear weak and dependent, moody, willpower and self-regulation ability, adaptability, control ability decline, etc., eager to be taken care of.

（3）Strong desire for help

Individuals who are in a state of illness all hope to get rid of the pain of the disease and strive for recovery. In order to reduce the suffering of pain and restore health as soon as possible, patients will actively seek help from others.

（4）Increased willingness to cooperate

Patients are eager to recover as soon as possible, so they will actively accept diagnosis, treatment and care, and actively and closely cooperate with medical workers, relatives and friends or other patients to strive for an early recovery.

（5）Obligations to assume social responsibilities before illness after recovery

After recovery, patients must step out of their role as patients and resume their original social roles to assume their original social responsibilities.

16.2.1.2　Difficulty adapting to the role of the patient

After an individual becomes ill, under normal circumstances, the patient will gradually adapt to the role of the patient, which is called role adaptation. However, there are still some patients who have difficulty changing from the previous social role to the patient role, or have difficulty changing from the patient role to the healthy person role during rehabilitation. These manifestations are called patient role adaptation difficulties. Common types are as follows.

（1）Patient's role conflict

Patient's role conflict refers to the incoordination of behavior caused by the psychological conflict between the patient and various roles before the disease because he is unable or unwilling to give up the original social role behavior when the role is changed. Patients often present with anxiety, anger, worry, confusion, and sadness. This situation is more common in people with more social or family responsibilities, and a strong sense of professionalism and responsibility.

（2）Patient's role reinforcement

After entering the patient's role, some patients show excessive identification with the disease state, and even feel fear and anxiety about the social role they will assume after the disease recovers, which is called patient role reinforcement. These patients are mainly manifested as being overly concerned about their diseases and over-relying on the hospital environment; after treatment improves or recovers, they are unwilling to change from the patient role to the normal role, often do not admit that the condition has improved or recovered, are unwilling to be discharged from the hospital, and are unwilling to leaving medical workers, unwilling to return to the original work, study and living environment.

（3）Absence of patient's role

Absence of patient's role means that patients are unaware of or have a negative attitude towards the disease, ignore the severity of their disease, refuse to act in the role of the patient, and some patients are eager to leave the role of the patient before they recover. Some people may be unprepared for a sudden illness, do not believe that they will get sick, and do not care; somepeople are too ignorant of the severity and consequences of the disease, or they are afraid to spend money because of financial stress, etc. The consequence may be rejection. Seeking medical treatment, delayed treatment, and further deterioration of the condition.

（4）Decreased patient's role

Patient's role decline refers to the fact that after the patient enters the patient's role, the disease has

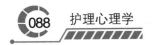

not yet been cured. For some reason, the patient quits the patient role prematurely and returns to the normal role in society, which is the opposite of role reinforcement. It is often due to emergencies at home or at work, such as a sudden illness of a relative, evaluation of work units, promotion of professional titles. Role decline usually occurs in the middle of the disease, and it is also a manifestation of the patient's role conflict, which is not conducive to further treatment and rehabilitation of the disease.

（5）Patient's role fear

Patient's role fear refers to the patient's lack of correct understanding and attitude towards the disease, and manifested as excessive worry, fear and other negative emotional responses to the disease after the disease, exaggerating the consequences of the disease, and lack of confidence in further treatment. Overly pessimistic and disappointed in recovery. They went to seek medical treatment everywhere, hoping to be freed from the disease immediately, so they went to the doctor in a hurry, and even abused drugs.

（6）Patient's role concealment

Patient's role concealment refers to the fact that the patient can not or will not bear the impact and consequences of the disease for some reason, so the truth of the disease is concealed. For example, AIDS patients and people with mental disorders keep their roles confidential, and patients hide their illnesses in order to comfort their families and avoid family worries.

（7）Patient's role impersonation

Patient's role impersonation means that there is no disease, but in order to escape certain social responsibilities and obligations or to obtain certain benefits, the patient pretends to be a patient role.

16.2.2　Psychological reactions of patients with malignant tumors

16.2.2.1　Shock and fear period

When the patient first learns of his malignant tumor, there will be a period of shock, which is called "diagnostic shock". The patient reacted strongly and strongly denied the diagnosis of malignant tumor, showing shock and fear, and some physical reactions such as palpitation, dizziness, fainting, and even stupor. This period is short, lasting a few days or a few questions.

16.2.2.2　Denial and dubt period

After the patient in the suspect stage calms down from the violent emotional reaction, he often uses the denial mechanism to protect himself. The patient begins to doubt whether the doctor's diagnosis is correct, and seeks medical treatment everywhere, hoping to find a doctor who can deny the diagnosis of malignant tumor, hoping for a miracle to happen; or do everything possible to explore the secrets of folk healing and adopt some unrealistic treatment options in order to survive.

16.2.2.3　Anger and depressed period

When patients gradually receive the diagnosis of malignant tumor, they will fall into extreme pain, and their emotions will become extremely fragile, irritable, angry, and sometimes accompanied by aggressive behavior; patients often feel sad, depression and even despair, and some patients even have suicidal thoughts or suicidal behavior.

16.2.2.4　Accept and adapt period

The fact that the patient is ill during the adaptation period can not be changed, and the patient can face the fact calmly, be calm, and cooperate with treatment. However, it is difficult for most patients to return to the state of mind before the disease, and they are often mildly depressed and anxious.

16.2.3 The role of nurses

(1) In clinical work, caregivers take care of patients, provide patients with direct nursing services, and meet the needs of patients in all aspects of physical, psychological and social aspects, which are the primary duties of nurses.

(2) Each nurse has management responsibilities. Nursing leaders manage human resources and material resources, organize the implementation of nursing work, and the purpose of management is to improve the quality and efficiency of nursing; general nurses manage patients and the ward environment to promote early recovery of patients.

(3) Nurses perform the function of educators on many occasions. In the hospital, educate the patients and their families about the treatment, nursing and prevention of diseases, and at the same time have the task of teaching and nursing students; in the community, educate the residents about the knowledge and methods of preventing diseases and maintaining health; in nursing schools, to impart professional knowledge and skills to nursing students.

(4) Protectors of patients' rights and interests. Nurses have the responsibility to help patients understand health information from various sources, supplement necessary information, and help patients make correct choices. Protect the rights and interests of patients from infringement and damage.

(5) Coordinators and collaborators. Nurses need to work closely with care recipients, families, and other health professionals to coordinate and support each other to better meet care recipients' needs.

(6) Nurses should play an exemplary role in preventive care, promotion of healthy lifestyles, etc. Such as do not smoke, pay attention to hygiene, strengthen physical exercise.

(7) Nurses have the responsibility to provide health information for nursing objects and give professional guidance such as preventive health care.

(8) Researchers carry out nursing research, solve complex clinical problems, and related problems encountered in nursing education, nursing management and other fields, improve nursing theory, and promote the development of nursing profession.

(9) Nursing reformers and entrepreneurs should adapt to the needs of social development, continuously reform the service mode of nursing, expand the scope and responsibilities of nursing, and promote the development of nursing.

Chapter 17 Disability

Summary

Objectives
1. Basic concept of disability.
2. Types of disability.
3. Mental response of the disabled.

Section 1 Overview

17.1.1 Concept of disability

Disability is any condition of the body ormind(impairment)that makes it more difficult for the person with the condition to do certain activities(activity limitation) and interact with the world around them (participation restrictions). Almost everyone is likely to experience some form of disability—temporary or permanent — at somepoint in life. Disabled people are also human beings, and they should also enjoy rights and dignity. The United Nations General Assembly will take December 3 every year as the international Day of Disabled People.

17.1.2 Caregivers learn the meaning of disability

Health care provider need to treat them equally as they have same need and same right for the treatment.

Need to be aware of how to effectively communicate with patients who have a range of disabilities, including people who are deaf or hard of hearing, or who have a speech, vision, or intellectual disability.

17.1.3 Classification of disability

People with disabilities are divided into six categories: physical disability, visual disability, hearing disability, intellectual disability, learning disability, mental disability.

17.1.3.1 Physical disability

Can be fluctuating or intermittent, chronic, progressive or stable, visible or invisible. Some involve extreme pain, some less, some none at all.

Progressive physical disability, e. g. , chronic arthritis, multiple sclerosis.

Non-progressive physical disability, e. g. , cerebral palsy, spina bifida.

17.1.3.2　Visual disability

Due to various reasons, the structure or function of visual organs or brain visual center is partially or completely affected, resulting in different degrees of visual loss or visual field reduction in both eyes, and visual function is difficult to be used freely and even lost when engaging in work, study or other activities like ordinary people. Only 10% of people are "legally blind". 90% have visual impairment. For example, color blind, cataract, glaucoma.

17.1.3.3　Hearing disability

Due to a variety of reasons lead to different degrees of permanent hearing impairment in both ears, can not hear or hear the sound of the surrounding environment or speech, as well as affect daily life and social participation. Ranges from hearing impairment to profound hearing loss.

17.1.3.4　Intellectual disability

Characterized by cognitive development and capacity that is significantly below average.

Involves a permanent limitation in a person's ability to learn. The causes of intellectual disability may be the influence of maternal illness during pregnancy, use of alcohol or drugs during pregnancy, genetics, childhood diseases.

17.1.3.5　Learning disability

A learning disability is essentially a specific and persistent disorder of a person's central nervous system affecting the learning process. This impacts a person's ability to either interpret what they see and hear, or to link information from different parts of the brain. Having a learning disability does not mean a person is incapable of learning; rather that they learn in a different way.

17.1.3.6　Mental disability

Mental disorder refers to the condition that all kinds of mental disorders have not been cured for more than one year, and there are cognitive, emotional and behavioral disorders, which affect daily life and activity participation. Schizophrenia accounts for the largest proportion of mental disabilities. Mental health disabilities can take many forms, just as physical disabilities do. Mood disorders—depression is the most common mood disorder. Anxiety disorders—phobias and panic disorder as well as obsessive—compulsive disorder. Eating disorders—anorexia nervosa and bulimia. Organic brain disorders—they are the result of physical disease or injury to the brain (e. g. , Alzheimer's disease, stroke, dementia).

17.1.4　Causes of disabilities

In addition to genetic causes of disabilities, there are many acquired causes, the main ones being trauma (brain or spinal cord injury), infection (encephalitis), exposure to harmful substances (carbon monoxide), emotional deprivation or lack of stimulation, and malnutrition.

Section 2　Mental Response of the Disabled

The onset of a chronic illness or disability typically triggers a chain of psychological reactions, which correspond to six phases of responses to physical disability.

(1) Ignorance period refers to a person after illness or physical function problems, don't know your

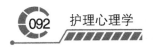

real condition, and don't realize the seriousness of the illness, not a long-term psychological ready to cope with illness and disability.

(2)Patients with shock refers to hear or conscious after the severity of the illness, the numbness in psychological or is a state of shock. The shock phase generally follows the period of ignorance and can last from a few seconds to a few days.

(3) Denies: patients in shock period of blow, in order to avoid their greater mental anguish, psychological deny the fact that have occurred.

(4)In patients with depression in the fully realized the severity of their condition and possible results, psychologically complete collapse, with their disease, and future life evaluation are more negative, sustained in a depressed emotional state. Periods of depression typically last for several months or longer.

(5)Against independent period after this refers to the patients with depression, mood have stabilized, but reverse in behavior, lack of positive independent living attitude and behavior.

(6)Adaptation: patients after the above stages, for their own psychological condition and prognosis are no longer worry overly, and able to take the initiative in the face of their disease and later life, actively cooperate with various treatment, the illness to their psychological basic adapted to the effects of stress.

Nurses must understand disability and how it affects people. Help patients, to meet the needs of patients, to provide comfort and quality care for patients with disabilities. In the process of care, nurses act as counselors, educators, negotiators and advocates for patients.

Counselor: provide emotional, intellectualand psychological support, listen to them, build rapport and therapeutic relationship with them.

Educator: provide adequate information when necessary.

Change agent: help patient to change behavior and lifestyle.

Nurses role/Intervention: provide modification to fulfill patient needs, e. g. , crutches, padded toilet seat, pictorial pain assessment chart for children.

Advocator: speak on behalf of patient.

Chapter 18　Hospitalization

Summary

> **Objectives**
> 1. Master the concept of hospitalization and the psychological nursing procedures.
> 2. Understand the psychological characteristics of hospitalized patients at different ages.
> 3. Understand the psychological care for emotional problems.

Section 1　Overview

18.1.1　Concept of hospitalization

The patient was admitted to hospital for treatment or observation.

18.1.2　Psychological nursing procedures

18.1.2.1　Psychological nursing evaluation

Psychological nursing evaluation is a comprehensive, systematic and in-depth objective description of the patient's mental state according to the theory and method of psychology. Scope of psychological nursing assessment. When assessing the existing or potential psychosocial problems of patients, nurses should first collect information. When the problems are found in which scope, the assessment can be focused on this scope, which is called focused assessment. For newly admitted patients, the initial psychological care assessment should include basic information, the patient's perception of health status, nutrition and metabolism, excretory function, level of volitional activity, sleep and rest, perception and cognition, self-cognition, role relationships, and ability to withstand stress.

18.1.2.2　Psychological nursing diagnosis

Psychological nursing diagnosis is based on the analysis of collected data on the basis of psychological assessment. So to determine the mental health problems of the nursing object and the causes of mental health problems is the basis for nurses to choose psychological nursing measures to achieve the expected results.

18.1.2.3　Psychological nursing plan

Psychological nursing plan is a specific psychological intervention measure which is formulated for the nursing problems raised by psychological nursing diagnosis. The contents and procedures of the plan should

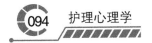

include the order of psychological nursing diagnosis; determine the desired goal; develop psychological nursing measures; the nursing plan is written.

18.1.2.4 Implementation of psychological nursing

The implementation of psychological nursing refers to the process of implementing psychological nursing plan and solving psychological problems of nursing objects in order to achieve the goal of psychological nursing. All proposed psycho – nursing diagnoses are resolved by implementing various psycho–nursing measures.

18.1.2.5 Psychological nursing evaluation

Psychological nursing evaluation is the identification and judgment of the cognitive, emotional and behavioral changes of patients after receiving psychological nursing. Nursing evaluation should run through the whole process of psychological nursing, and should be adjusted according to the evaluation results.

Section 2 Psychological Characteristics of Hospitalized Patients at Different Ages

18.2.1 Psychological characteristics of children patients

(1) Hospitalized children with separation anxiety, away from their main caregivers and familiar environment, will first appear "separation anxiety", manifested as anxiety, often crying, refusing to eat, not taking medicine, sleep restlessness, coupled with the strange hospital environment, other children's crying, will aggravate the anxiety of children.

(2) Fear, resistance is also one of the main manifestations of children. Fear is associated with the removal of children from their parents and familiar environment in hospital, lack of knowledge about medical procedures and being forced to undergo some procedures. Under the influence of strong fear, some children will refuse to be hospitalized, refuse to receive treatment, or shout, break things and other performance: some children to visit the parents silence, resist, ignore, in order to express their unhappy mood.

(3) Skin hunger. Human beings, like all warm–blooded animals, have a special need to touch and touch each other, this phenomenon is called "skin hunger". Parent – child touch is a very important psychological need for infants. When young hospitalized children leave their mothers, this special need cannot be met, which is often manifested as crying, lack of appetite, sleep restlessness and so on.

(4) Pain and suffering caused by behavioral degenerative diseases, coupled with anxiety and fear caused by hospitalization, may lead to behavioral degradation of children, such as bed–wetting, acting in pettish, refusing to eat, crying before bed, passive dependence.

18.2.2 Psychological characteristics of young patients

The psychological characteristics of young people are rapidly to mature but not mature, which determines that young patients in the face of disease mood is often changeable, with obvious polarity, easy to move from one extreme to the other extreme.

18.2.2.1 Shock and denial

Young people are full of infinite longing and yearning for life and the future. At this time, when you know that you have a disease, especially a serious disease, you will first be shocked, difficult to accept, and then do not believe the doctor's diagnosis, the performance of "denial", deny your disease, it is difficult to enter the role of a patient, refuse to accept treatment. It is only when you really feel the pain and physical weakness that you gradually accept the fact that you are ill.

18.2.2.2   Anxiety and impatience

Young people often worry that disease will bring adverse effects on study, work, love, marriage and so on, showing anxiety. The treatment is often impatient and impatient, hoping for a quick fix. Once the treatment fails to achieve the desired effect, or the disease repeats, they show impatience. When the condition is getting better, they are often blindly optimistic and do not take medication according to the doctor's advice and do not cooperate with treatment.

18.2.2.3   Pessimism and disappointment

When the disease enters the chronic phase or leaves sequelae or even worsens, it will cause a great blow to young people, prone to depression, pessimism, disappointment and even depression. Young people are prone to extreme psychological and behavioral behavior, self-abandonment, abandonment of treatment, and even suicidal thoughts.

18.2.2.4   Loneliness and loneliness

After hospitalization, young people leave the familiar family, school, classmates and partners, live in a strange hospital, can only silently bear the pain of the disease, lead a monotonous and boring life. A little longer hospital stay will appear lonely, lonely, bored and other emotions.

18.2.3   Psychological characteristics of middle-aged patients

Middle-aged patients play an important role in family and society, their personality and emotions are relatively stable, but once they fall ill, they often show complex psychological activities.

18.2.3.1   Anxiety and impatience

Middle-aged people are more prone to anxiety after illness because of their important family and social roles. Anxiety will lead to its disease treatment in the show of impatient mood, and can not rest assured, hope to be cured as soon as possible, as soon as possible, some patients will give up their own health for various reasons, interrupt treatment, early discharge.

18.2.3.2   Pessimism and depression

Middle-aged peoplecan not work normally after illness, the reduction of economic sources, coupled with expensive medical expenses, as well as the problems of supporting parents and children's education, so that they have pessimism and disappointment, feel a strong sense of helplessness and hopelessness, and even have the idea of suicide, in order to reduce the financial burden of the family or escape their inner suffering.

18.2.3.3   Menopause syndrome

Middle-aged people in physical strength and energy began to transition to the elderly, often appear physical and energy poor performance, this time disease, will accelerate this transition, can appear menopause syndrome. Accompanied by obvious symptoms of autonomic nervous disorder, such as headache, dizziness, insomnia, lack of appetite, palpitation shortness of breath, fear of cold and heat.

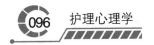

18.2.4 Psychological characteristics of elderly patients

18.2.4.1 Strong self-esteem

The elderly have strong self-esteem and hope to get the respect and compliment of doctors and nurses. Unwillingness to take orders, especially from young medical staff. Sometimes they even suddenly refuse treatment and care, and sometimes they are aggressive and do things they can't do, such as going to the toilet alone, walking without help, sticking to their original eating habits, which can easily lead to some accidents.

18.2.4.2 Inferiority and depression

The decline of the social and family status of the elderly, as well as the gradual decline of the body, often leads to inferiority. Once sick, often feel that their days on earth are not long, many want to do things can not be completed, further aggravating the sense of inferiority and worthlessness. The elderly often suffer from chronic or aging diseases, and often lack confidence in the recovery of the disease, self-pity, and then produce depression, so it is not uncommon for the elderly to commit suicide.

18.2.4.3 Fear and loneliness

When the illness is more serious, the elderly are often aware of the approach of death, so they show emotional reactions such as fear of death and fear. Some of these emotions are expressed in words, but many are hidden in the heart. The elderly fear loneliness, especially when they are ill, and crave the comfort, care and companionship of others.

18.2.4.4 Self-centered

Some elderly people stereotype, stubborn, often self-centered, sick and hospitalized often require medical staff diagnosis and treatment work, in line with their own life order and habits: often ask family members to pay more attention to their own, over-dependence on family.

18.2.4.5 Degenerate

Some elderly people become naive after illness emotion and behavior, often put forward unrealistic requirements, mood swings, poor self-control, often conflict with family members, patients, medical staff. Some elderly people are not willing to be discharged from hospital, dependent on medical staff and family members, and need others to help them do what they can. Even like children, there is the phenomenon of "old children".

18.2.4.6 Avoid

In order to avoid mental pressure, some elderly patients avoid events or topics related to the disease for a long time. When they are alone, they often shed tears and hide their inner feelings.

Section 3   Emotional Problems of Psychological Nursing

Anxiety, depression, fear and anger are the main emotional problems that often occur in patients after illness.

18.3.1　Anxiety

18.3.1.1　Definition of anxiety

Anxiety refers to an unpleasant emotional experience experienced by patients when they are faced with an unclear, vague or imminent threat or danger. It is commonly seen in the following patients: children or elderly patients, patients newly admitted and admitted to the ICU, patients undergoing surgery, and patients undergoing other special or invasive diagnostic and nursing measures.

18.3.1.2　Psychological nursing for anxiety

(1) Establish a good nurse – patient relationship: the establishment of a good nurse – patient relationship has an important impact on the effect of psychological nursing, requiring nurses in the implementation of psychological nursing process, always put a good nurse–patient relationship in the first place, and throughout the psychological nursing process.

(2) Provide appropriate support: the support that nurses can provide to patients includes information support, emotional support and social support. Information support refers to all kinds of knowledge needed by patients, such as hospital rules and regulations, disease diagnosis, treatment, prognosis and other related knowledge.

(3) Techniques of psychological counseling and therapy: ① relaxation therapy; ② systematic desensitization therapy; ③ biofeedback therapy; ④ rational emotive behavior therapy.

(4) psychotropic drug treatment: patients with serious anxiety can be advised to consult a psychiatric department for psychological treatment or drug treatment.

18.3.2　Depression

18.3.2.1　Definition of depression

Depression is characterized by low mood, slow thinking, loss of interest, feeling that life is meaningless, hopeless and depressed, and even suicidal thoughts or behaviors in serious cases. Depression is common in patients who are seriously ill, chronically ill and elderly.

18.3.2.2　Psychological nursing for depression

According to the results of evaluation and the level of psychological problems, combined with the specific clinical situation to choose appropriate psychological nursing technology to implement psychological nursing for patients.

(1) Good nurse–patient relationship.

(2) Actively seek social support: patients are encouraged to talk to relatives, friends and medical staff to seek more social support.

(3) Psychological counseling and treatment techniques: ① rational emotive behavior therapy; ② family therapy; ③ relaxation therapy; ④ urge sleep therapy.

(4) Actively participate in social activities: when the patient is in a state of depression, he can be encouraged to do as his physical condition allows take part in a variety of social activities to divert attention from illness and physical symptoms.

(5) Psychological treatment or psychotropic drug treatment: patients with serious depression can be advised to consult a psychiatric department for psychological treatment or drug treatment.

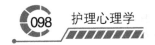

18.3.3　Fear

18.3.3.1　Definition of fear

Fear is a psychological experience that occurs when a patient is faced with a specific and definite threat or danger. Clinically, fear is most common in children and surgical patients. Factors that cause fear include the special atmosphere and environment of the hospital, the threat of disease, certain dangerous or invasive examinations, surgery, and diseases with poor prognosis or life-threatening conditions.

18.3.3.2　Psychological nursing of fear

(1) Eliminate the object and cause of fear: the nurse should analyze and confirm the cause and situation of the patient's fear. Before the patient's fear, the nurse should take the initiative to explain the pain and threat that may be brought to the patient appropriately, so as to weaken or eliminate the dangerous situation, and give the patient appropriate hints and guarantees.

(2) Psychological counseling and treatment techniques: ①model law; ②positive reinforcement method; ③relaxation therapy; ④rational emotive behavior therapy; ⑤systematic desensitization therapy helps patients relax from the low level of fear until they can face the most fearful situation; ⑥catharsis.

18.3.4　Anger

18.3.4.1　Definition of anger

Anger is an emotional experience that occurs when a person's needs can not be met, desires can not be realized, and obstacles or setbacks occur in the pursuit of a certain goal.

18.3.4.2　Psychological nursing of anger

Due to the particularity of medical industry, medical staff often encounter various situations of patients' anger in their work. Angry emotions of patients will not only reduce their cooperation in treatment and nursing and trust of medical staff, affect the treatment of diseases, but also easily deepen the contradiction between doctors and patients, cause medical disputes, and seriously damage the image of hospitals and medical staff. Effective communication with angry patients and good psychological care are particularly important in today's medical environment.

(1) Understand and accept the patient's anger: ask at least 3 other "seemingly nonsense" questions that may have nothing to do with the core situation of diagnosis and treatment, so that the patient can answer "Yes", so that the patient can agree with the nurse's questions. For example, the nurse can ask "Do you feel abdominal pain?" "You want relief as soon as possible?" "Are you in a hurry?" This kind of questioning can help the patient feel understood and accepted, laying the foundation for further communication.

(2) Change the environment: after the patient is emotionally stable, find an environment conducive to communication, such as a quiet and comfortable office or conference room, and get away from the situation and characters that cause the patient's anger. At the same time, self-protection measures should be taken. There should be no harmful objects in the communication environment, such as knives, glass instruments; fixed stool should be used, and the nurse should sit near the door.

(3) Psychological counseling and treatment techniques: ① emotional catharsis; ② supportive psychological intervention; ③relaxation therapy.

Chapter 19　Loss and Grief

Objectives
1. Definition of loss.
2. Defination of greif.
3. Understanding the impact of loss and grief in healthcare settings.

Section 1　Loss

19.1.1　Definition of loss

The fact or process of losing something or someone. Occurred when someone or something can no longer be seen, heard, known, felt or experienced.

The loss, through death, of loved ones (bereavement) can occur at any stage of the life cycle (a non-normative influence). However, it becomes more likely as we get older. Some losses are more "non-normative" than others, such as the loss of a child. This can occur at any stage from conception through to childhood and adolescence, and beyond. Miscarriage, stillbirth and neonatal death are all forms of bereavement, as are terminations.

The psychological and bodily reactions that occur in people who suffer bereavement (whatever form it takes) are called grief. The "observable expression of grief" is called mourning, although this term is often used to refer to the social conventions surrounding death (such as funerals and wearing black clothes).

But grief can "begin" before the actual death, and those who are dying can also grieve for their own death. Nurses have a crucial role to play in helping patients with a terminal illness to accept their condition. They're in the privileged position of being able to listen to patients talking about their hopes and fears, and their experience, knowledge and skills may enable patients to explore their feelings and come to terms with their condition. The patients may be children, adolescents or adults.

Examples of losses are shown in Table 19-1.

Table 19-1　Examples of losses

Losses	Example
Familiar environment	Earthquake
A part of the self	Body part (amputee) or function (hearing loss) or self-esteem (being sacked by employer)

Continued to Table 19-1

Losses	Example
Independence	Prison
Relationship	Divorce
Financial security	Bankrupt
Social status	Refugees
A loved being	Parents or pets

19.1.2 Type of loss

(1)Sudden loss:unexpected accident,heart attack.

(2)Gradual loss:gradual deterioration,involve aging and chronic disease.

(3)Anticipated loss:expected and predictable progression.

(4)Uncertain loss:some diseases have high degree of uncertainty (infectious diseases).

(5)Overall loss:death of a loved one,terminal illness.

(6)Partial loss:false away part of the sickness and disability,e. g. ,mosteitomy.

(7)Permanet loss:no hope of recovery,such as kidney failure.

(8)Temporary loss:good hope for recovery,such as a denoma.

Section 2   Grief

19.2.1 Definition of grief

Grief is a natural response to loss. Grieving is a normal reaction that helps a person to recover slowly from the loss. The process of grieving for a dying person before death (anticipatory grief) is a process of "letting go".

Grief has been variously depicted as follows:(a)a natural human reaction,(b)a psychiatric disorder, (c) a disease process.

All three approaches contain an element of truth. As far as (a) is concerned,grief is a universal feature of human existence,found in all cultures. But its form and the intensity of its expression vary considerably. As far as (b) is concerned,although grief itself has never been classified as a mental disorder,the psychiatric framework emphasizes the human suffering grief involves, and therefore provides a useful balance to viewing it simply as a natural reaction.

Regarding (c),although there may be increased rates of morbidity (health deterioration) or mortality (death) among bereaved people,these aren't necessarily directly caused by the grief process. For example, the effects of change in lifestyle (such as altered nutrition or drug intake),or increased attention to physical illness,which predated the bereavement,might be mistaken for the effects of grief itself. However, there's substantial evidence that bereaved spouses are more at risk of dying themselves compared with matched non-bereaved controls. This is true mainly for widowers,and especially for younger widowers experiencing an unexpected bereavement.

Acute grieve is a reaction that begins at the time of a loss, e. g. , loss of a limb as the result of an accident. All individuals do not grief in exactly the same way. Periods of grieving varies.

19.2.2 Types of grief

(1) Anticipatory. Before actual loss, e. g. , for family caregivers, grieving can start long before the person you are caring for passes way.

(2) Acute. At time of loss.

(3) Chronic. Grief that lasts over an extended period of time and can be intermittent, e. g. , parents with disabled child.

(4) Delayed. Postponed until a later time, e. g. , a wife putting it off death of husband because need to attend to children first.

(5) Suppressed. It is repressed/restrained for years, and need the trigger factor, e. g. , a mother suffer miscarriage now but suppressed her grief but only show later in an excessive manner when her own daughter suffers miscarriage.

19.2.3 Stages of grieving

Every person does not necessarily experience all the stages nor does a person necessarily experience them is any precise order.

Kubler-Ross's stage account was based on her pioneering work with over 200 terminally ill patients. She was interested in how they prepared for their imminent deaths (anticipatory grief), and so her stages describe the process of dying. But she was inspired by an earlier version of Bowlby's theory and her stages were later applied (by other researchers) to grief for others. Her theory remains very influential in nursing and counselling, with both dying patients and the bereaved.

(1) Denial and isolation

This stage is accompanied by thoughts such as "this can not be happening to me" "it's not true". The person emotionally denies the loss that has occurred or is about to occur. Commonly withdraw from social interactions and may seek the opinion of several other doctors, traditional remedies, hoping the initial diagnosis was incorrect. This prevents the patient from being overwhelmed by the initial shock. It may take the form of seeking a second opinion, or holding contradictory beliefs. Denial (or, at least, partial denial) is used by most patients not only at this early stageof their illness, but also later on. It's as if they can contemplate the possibility of their own death for a defined time period, but then have to turn away from such thoughts so that they can carry on with life. Denial acts as a buffer system, allowing the patient time to develop other coping mechanisms. It can also bring isolation. The patient may fear rejection and abandonment in suffering and feel that nobody understands what the suffering is like. Avoidance by staff, for whatever reasons, can exacerbate this feeling of isolation in terminal illness.

Almost all the patients she interviewed initially denied they had life-threatening illnesses, although only three remained in a constant state of denial (the rest drifted in and out). Denial was more common when someone had been given the diagnosis in an abrupt or insensitive way, or if they were surrounded by family and(or) staff who were also in denial. Searching for a second opinion was a very common initial reaction, representing a desperate attempt to change the unpredictable world they'd just been catapulted into, back into the world they knew and understood.

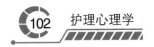

（2）Anger

The person begins to realize that the loss and experience thoughts such as "Why me? why is this happening? why now?" He may experience anger, frustration as he begins to realize that nothing can be done to change the situation. This may be directed at doctors, nurses, relatives, other healthy people who'll go on living. This can be the most difficult stage for family and staff to deal with. They may react personally to the patient's anger and respond with anger of their own; this only increases the patient's hostile behaviour.

（3）Bargaining

Occurs when the person tries to postpone reality by making a "deal", e. g. , with fate. This is an attempt to postpone death by "doing a deal" with fate(or the hospital), much as a child might bargain with its parents in order to get its own way. So, it has to include a prize for "good behaviour" and sets a self-imposed "deadline" such as a son or daughter's wedding; the patient promises not to ask for more time if this postponement is granted.

（4）Depression

He may experience depression, as he begins to realize that nothing can be done to alter the situation. This is likely to arise when the patient realizes that no bargain can be struck and that death is inevitable. She/he grieves for all the losses that death represents. This is preparatory depression, a form of preparatory grief that helps the patient to prepare him/herself for the final separation from the world. Reactive depression involves expressions of fear and anxiety and a sense of great loss of body image, job, financial security, or ability to continue caring for children. Depression is a common reaction in the dying. For example, Hinton (1975) reported that 18% of those who committed suicide suffered from serious physical illnesses, with 4% having illnesses that probably would have killed them within 6 months. Elderly people who've lived full lives have relatively little to grieve for—they've gained much and lost few opportunities. But people who perceive lives full of mistakes and missed opportunities may, paradoxically, have more to grieve for as they begin to realize that these opportunities are now lost for ever. This resembles Erikson's despair, as does resignation, which Kübler–Ross distinguished from acceptance. The detachment and stillness of those who've achieved acceptance comes from calmness, while in those who've become resigned it comes from despair. The latter can not accept death, nor can they deny its existence any longer. Kübler–Ross found that there are a few patients who fight to the end, struggle and keep hoping, which makes it almost impossible for them to achieve true acceptance.

（5）Acceptance

The person may realize the inevitability of the situation and accepts the loss. He is either depressed or angry about his fate and is able to talk about his loss. Almost devoid of feelings, the patient seems to have given up the struggle for life, sleeps more and withdraws from other people, as if preparing for "the long journey". Hope (for a cure, a new drug or a miracle) is the constant thread running through all these stages and is necessary to maintain the patient's morale through the illness. Hope is rationalisation of suffering for some and a means of much–needed denial for others. Kübler Ross found that if a patient stopped expressing hope, it was usually a sign of imminent death.

19.2.4　Assisting the grieving persons

Total absence of grief , not a healthy sign and unresolved grief can lead to delayed or distorted reactions. The grieving person may experience a wide range of feelings: shock, anger, sadness, guilt, depression, despair, relief, hope, and acceptance. Expression of feelings may include crying, withdraw from people, lack of energy, not motivated, hostile behaviour, physical symptoms, e. g. , inability to sleep, to eat, chest pain, headaches, gastrointestinal disturbances. The person must be allowed and encouraged to work through his grief, encourage expression of feelings by listening. According to March, "Most nurses are confronted with the reality of death with a regularity that lay people would find shocking..." Dying is a major crisis, which can be painfully distressing, unfamiliar and frightening. In order to help patients and their families through this process, nurses need to develop awareness of their own attitudes and ability to face terminal illness and death, and their particular prejudices and convictions.

Section 3　Lose and Greif in Medical Condition

19.3.1　Communicating with dying adult patients

Research suggests that a proportion of patients don't wish to talk about the terminal nature of their condition. They may cope by avoiding having to focus on their prognosis, or seeking escape in light hearted conversation. In spite of these findings, authors have urged nurses, as a kind of blanket rule of good communication, to discuss with patients their feelings about their prognosis.

Dean proposes that nurses develop communication skills that not only allow them to talk sensitively about death and dying with patients but also give them the capacity to assess whether or not this is what the patient wants. Similarly, Parkinson maintains that providing opportunities to talk with patients so that they can express their fears, anger or depression should comprise a major focus of the nurse's work.

Webster observed nurses communicating with dying patients in four English hospitals. They often displayed "blocking" behaviour, avoiding intimate conversations by changing the subject, ignoring cues, making jokes or tailoring their responses to the least distressing aspect of the issues raised. Such light-hearted interactions allowed the nurses to sidestep potentially difficult conversations, keeping them on emotional "safe ground". Wilkinson (1991, in Dean) observed similar behaviour in 54 cancer nurses. Their blocking behaviours predominated over facilitative behaviours. For example, the psychosexual impact that gynecological, bladder or bowel malignancy may have had on patients' lives was never discussed during the observed interactions. This was confirmed by Costello.

According to Hare and Pratt, until recently a death on the ward was a violent reminder of the failings of nursing/medicine. But major developments, such as growth of the hospice movement, suggest that the emphasis is changing from curing to caring. March maintains that "Nursing appears to be redefining itself to include the whole hearted care of dying and bereaved people..." Western culture generally has been moving since the 1960s towards open communication about death and dying, with paternalistic notions that patients would be too upset to discuss death slowly changing.

19.3.2　Communicating with dying child patients

Children with a life-threatening illness sense that it's serious and that they might die or are dying, even if they're not explicitly told. Their anxiety levels are markedly higher than those of chronically ill children, even if undergoing the same number and duration of treatments. This anxiety and sense of isolation persists when the child isn't in hospital and even during periods of remission in children with Leukemia.

The hospitalized dying child's awareness of death is more sharply focused when another child dies on the ward. If the child has the same illness, the link between that event and the dying child's imminent death is made more immediate. Judd believes that there's a more open and honest attitude on children's wards in most hospitals, where death and dying are often discussed openly in response to parents' questions and sometimes with the children, depending on the ethos of the unit.

Effective communication with dying children will be influenced by nurses' values, attitudes and beliefs, which in turn are influenced by past experience and religious, cultural and societal beliefs. Chesterfield cites studies showing that doctors and nurses become skilled at withdrawal and distancing techniques; these strategies may help protect the practitioner from distress but inhibit effective communication with the dying child. The family may not want the child's impending death discussed openly, shielding the child from distress or because of their own fears. This mutual pretence—Kübler-Ross's mutual pretence awareness (see above)—can prove functional in maintaining hope and the roles of individual family members.

Clearly, the dying child needs an age- and developmentally appropriate opportunity to share its fears and concerns. This doesn't mean imposing a discussion, but involves attempting to be open to the child's willingness (or otherwise) to talk. If the child seems to be "somewhere else" emotionally—but not depressed—this may be a very understandable way of achieving separation from the world around them. This should be tolerated and respected, rather than pressurizing the child to be jolly or "hang on" for the sake of others. As Judd points out, this choosing to withdraw may be the one area of control the child has left.

19.3.3　Death in accdent and emergency departments

The news of death can provoke an alarm reaction: the world suddenly becomes a threatening, unpredictable place. Anything that makes the loss unreal (such as a sudden, unexpected death and/or one that occurs in unusual or violent circumstances) is likely to make it more difficult to accept, which can produce a more prolonged and complicated grief reaction. Nurses in accdent and emergency (A&E) are likely to have to deal with a higher proportion of such deaths than those working in other areas. Indeed, one-third of all deaths in hospital occur within the first few hours of a patient's arrival.

According to Smith, although the hospice and palliative care movements have done much to prepare nurses as well as patients for death and for the terminal phase of conditions such as cancer and AIDS, many nurses in acute care still feel unprepared and unsupported. We live in a society where cardiovascular disease and accidents are majorcauses of mortality, and these deaths tend to occur in hospital with little or no warning for staff, let alone relatives or friends.

Wright has looked at the issue of nurses coping with sudden death in A&E (and ICU, coronary care unit and pediatric ICU) in the USA. He concluded that the best mental health outcomes for relatives and staff depended on the foundations laid at the time of the patient's arrival in A&E. He now runs crisis training, education and counselling (CRI-TEC), a support service in the UK for those affected by sudden death. It provides courses for health professionals, the police and the fire brigade.

Staff caring for the newly bereaved should be able to provide support early on and help build a foundation for the relatives' recovery process. But nursing and medical staff often feel inadequately prepared to meet relatives' needs. In A&E the situation is complicated by the fact that staff and relatives meet at a time of crisis, the meeting is usually brief, unexpected and may not have any follow-up. In contrast, a ward environment often allows time for a relationship and rapport to develop. The ethos of A&E is to save life, so when the patient dies this often leads to feelings of failure. But the input of highly trained and motivated nursing and medical staff, who understand the importance of bereavement care, can help relatives' psychological recovery.

Summary

Objectives

1. Define death and dying.
2. Understand the stages of death.
3. Understand the impact on family members.
4. Learn about end-of-life care.

Section 1   Near Death and Dying

20.1.1   Concept

20.1.1.1   Definition of near death

After a patient has received therapeutic or palliative care, his or her condition, although he or she is clearly conscious, deteriorates at an accelerated rate, indicating that the end of life is near. So dying is the last stage of life.

20.1.1.2   Definition of death

Death is the disintegration of the integrity of the organism, the cessation of the metabolic process in the body, that is, the end of human life activities, that is, the permanent termination of individual life functions.

20.1.2   Death standard

20.1.2.1   Traditional death criteria

Cardiac arrest and respiratory arrest have been used as criteria for death for thousands of years.

20.1.2.2   Criteria for brain death

At present, the medical profession proposes a new objective standard, which is the standard of brain death. Brain death is total brain death, including the irreversible death of the brain, midbrain, cerebellum and brainstem. Irreversible brain death is a symbol of the end of life. The standard of brain death proposed by Harvard University in 1968 are as follows.

(1) No sensitivity and reactivity.

(2) No movement, no breathing.

(3) No reflection.

（4）Flat brain waves.

The diagnosis of brain death can be made after repeated review within 24 hours without any change in the above criteria and excluding the influence of body temperature below 32 ℃ and central nervous system inhibitors.

20.1.3　Stages of the death process

Death does not occur suddenly, but is a progressive process, generally divided into three stages.

20.1.3.1　Near death

The near death period, also known as the terminal state, is the beginning of the process of dying. During this period, the functions of various systems in the body are extremely weak, and the functions of the parts above the king of the brain in the central nervous system are in a state of deep inhibition, showing blurred or loss of consciousness, weakened or dull reflex, hypotonia or disappearance of muscle, weakened heartbeat, decreased blood pressure, weak breathing or tidal breathing and intermittent breathing. The duration of the near-death period may vary with the physical condition of the patient and the cause of death. Patients such as sudden death may enter the clinical death period directly. This period of life in a reversible stage, timely and effective rescue treatment, life can be revived; otherwise, it enters the stage of clinical death.

20.1.3.2　Clinical death

In the stage of clinical death, the inhibitory process of the central nervous system has spread from the cerebral cortex to the subcortical area, and the medulla oblongata is in a state of extreme inhibition. The performance is heartbeat, breathing completely stopped, pupil dilated, all kinds of reflex disappeared, but all kinds of tissue cells still have weak and short metabolic activities. This period usually lasts five to six minutes, beyond which irreversible changes will occur in the brain. However, under low temperature conditions, especially when the head is cooled and brain oxygen consumption is reduced, the clinical death period can be extended to 1 hour or more.

20.1.3.3　Biological death

The biological death stage is the final stage of the death process. During this period, the metabolism of the whole central nervous system and various organs stopped successively, and irreversible changes occurred. The whole body could not be revived. With the progress of this period, the early cadaver phenomenon appeared successively, namely corpse cold, lividity, mortis and so on; the late cadaver phenomenon, namely corpse corruption and so on.

Section 2　Hospice Care

20.2.1　Concept of hospice care

Care is also known as good death services: hospice care, resting place, etc. Hospice care is to provide a comprehensive care for terminally ill patients and their families, including physical, psychological, social and other aspects, so that the terminally ill patient's life is respected, the symptoms are controlled, the quality of life is improved, the physical and mental health of the family members are maintained and

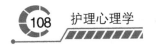

enhanced, so that the patient can finish the final journey of life without pain, peace and comfort at the end of life.

20.2.2　Development of hospice care

Modern hospice care was founded in the 1960s. In 1976, the founder Dr. Sanders established the world's first "St. Christopher's Hospice Hospital" in Britain, which was praised as "The beacon of the hospice movement in the world". Since then, more than 60 countries, including the U. S. , France, Japan and Canada, have provided hospice care services. In July 1988, Tianjin Medical College, funded by Dr. HuangTianzhong, a Chinese American, established the first hospice care research center in China. In October of the same year, Nanhui Nursing Home, the first hospice hospital in China, was born in Shanghai. All these indicate that our country has entered the ranks of the world hospice care research and practice. Since then, many provinces such as Shenyang, Beijing and Nanjing have launched hospice care services and established hospice care institutions.

20.2.3　Research object of hospice care

Hospice care is not only a kind of service, but also a kind of research object to explore the physiological and psychological development of terminally ill patients and to provide comprehensive care for the terminally ill patients and reduce the mental pressure of the patients' families. It is a new frontier discipline closely related to medicine, nursing science, sociology, psychology, ethics, health economics, policy science, law and other disciplines.

20.2.4　Organizational form and concept of dying patients

20.2.4.1　Organization form of hospice care

(1)Specialized hospice care institutions.

(2)General hospitals are equipped with hospice wards.

(3)Home care.

20.2.4.2　Principle of hospice care

(1)Transition from treatment-oriented treatment to treatment-oriented care: hospice care is aimed at the terminal stage of various diseases, advanced tumors, treatment is no longer effective, life is about to end, for these patients not through treatment to avoid death, but through comprehensive physical and mental care, provide moderate, palliative treatment for dying patients, control symptoms, relieve pain, eliminate anxiety, fear, obtain psychological and social support, so that they get the final peace.

(2) To extend the survival time of patients into improving the quality of life of patients: hospice care does not focus on prolonging the survival time, but aims to enrich the limited life of patients and improve the quality of life in the terminal stage. It provides a comfortable, meaningful, dignified and hopeful life for terminal patients, so that patients can have a clear mind in the limited time, receive care in controllable pain, and enjoy the last journey of life.

(3)Respect for the dignity and rights of the terminally ill patient: the terminally ill patient is a person who is near death but not yet dead. As long as he is not in a coma, he still has thoughts, consciousness, feelings and personal dignity and rights. Medical staff should pay attention to the maintenance and maintenance of human value and dignity, in the end-of-life care should allow patients to retain their original lifestyle, try to meet their reasonable requirements, retain the right to personal privacy, participate in the formulation of medical care plan.

(4) Pay attention to the psychological support of terminally ill patients' families: while providing comprehensive care for terminally ill patients, we also provide psychological and social support for terminally ill patients' families, so as to gain the strength to accept the death of their loved ones and calmly face death. So that the patient's family can provide services for the patient while he was alive and provide funeral services after his death.

Section 3   Nursing of Dying Patients

20.3.1   Physiological changes

(1) Sensory perception and consciousness changes are manifested as gradual loss of vision and disappearance of vision. Dry eyes, increased secretions, dilated pupils, hearing is often the last of the human body to disappear a feeling. Changes in consciousness can be manifested as drowsiness, confusion, lethargy, coma, etc.

(2) Loss of muscle tone is manifested as urinary and stool incontinence, difficulty swallowing, inability to maintain a good and comfortable functional position, weakness of the limbs, inability to carry out independent physical activities, facial appearance changes to theHsi face, namely, slightly thin facial muscle, lead gray face, sunken eyes, eyes half open, jaw droop, mouth slightly open, etc.

(3) The gradual weakening of gastrointestinal peristalsis is manifested as loss of appetite, abdominal distension, nausea, vomiting, constipation, dehydration, dry mouth, etc.

(4) Circulation capacity loss is manifested as pale skin, wet cold, a lot of sweating, limbs cyanosis, spots, pulse fast and weak, irregular or undetectable, blood pressure reduction or undetectable, apex pulsation is often the last to disappear.

(5) Respiratory dysfunction is manifested as respiratory rate changes from fast to slow, respiratory depth changes from deep to shallow, nasal respiration, tidal respiration, open mouth respiration, and finally respiratory arrest. Sputum and snore breathing may occur.

(6) Pain manifests as restlessness, changes in blood pressure and heart rate, faster or slower breathing, unusual posture, and painful face. Such as twisted features, frowning, eyes open or closed, eyes distracted, teeth clenched.

(7) Near death signs of various reflexes gradually disappear, dystonia, loss, rapid and weak pulse, decreased blood pressure, shortness of breath, difficulty, damp breathing, skin cold. Usually breathing stops first, followed by cardiac arrest. Sudden death often results in cardiac arrest.

20.3.2   Nursing measures

20.3.2.1   Promote patient comfort

(1) Maintain a good and comfortable position and strengthen skin care.

(2) Attach importance to oral care, assist patients with gargling in the morning, after meals and before

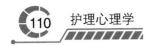

going to bed, and maintain oral cleanliness.

20.3.2.2 Nutritional support to obtain psychological support

(1) Take the initiative to explain the cause of digestive symptoms to patients and family members to reduce anxiety.

(2) Pay attention to the color, aroma and taste of food, eat a smallamount of meals to reduce nausea and increase appetite.

(3) Give liquid or semi-liquid diet that is easy for the patient to swallow. If necessary, nasal feeding or complete parenteral nutrition should be used to ensure the nutritional supply of patients.

(4) Strengthen monitoring, observe the patient's electrolyte index and nutritional status.

20.3.2.3 Promote blood circulation

(1) Observe the patient's vital signs, skin color and temperature.

(2) When the limbs of the patient are cold and uncomfortable, they should strengthen the warmth, and give the hot waterbag when necessary, but the water temperature should not exceed 50 ℃.

(3) Pay attention to clean and dry skin.

20.3.2.4 Improve respiratory function

(1) Keep the indoor air fresh and ventilate regularly.

(2) For conscious patients, the semi-decubitus position is adopted to expand the chest volume, reduce the amount of blood return to the heart and improve dyspnea. For comatose patients, the supine position with the head tilted to one side or side is adopted to prevent respiratory secretions from straying into the trachea and causing asphyxia or pulmonary complications.

(3) When necessary, use suction device to suck out sputum and maintain airway patency.

(4) According to the degree of dyspnea to give oxygen, correct the state of hypoxia, improve respiratory function.

20.3.2.5 Reduce sensory and perceptual stimuli

(1) To provide quiet, fresh air, good ventilation, acertain warmth facilities, appropriate lighting environment, to avoid patients because of blurred vision fear, fear psychology, increase the sense of security.

(2) Timely wipe eye secretions with wet gauze, patients can apply eye ointment such as holomycin or vaseline gauze when the eyelid can not be closed, in order to protect the cornea, prevent cornea dry ulcer or conjunctivitis.

(3) Nursing should prevent whispering around the patient, so as not to increase the patient's anxiety. Can be used to touch the patient and other non-verbal communication, with a soft and gentle tone of voice, clear.

Chapter 21　Stress Management

Summary

Objectives

1. Grasp the meaning of pressure and pressure source.
2. Familiar different kinds of pressure sources.
3. Understand the impact of stress on the body and learn ways to cope with stress.

Section 1　Overview of Stress and Stressful Events

21.1.1　Overview of stress

20.1.1.1　Concept of stress

Any type of change that causes physical, emotional or psychological strain in an individual. Any change in life or habit can be called stress. It's the body's response to anything that requires attention or action.

20.1.1.2　Sources of stress

Any factor that causes stress and reduces stress. For example, changes from emotional, physical, social or economic aspects.

Accurate identification of stressors helps predict stress, and most people are able to respond more effectively to stress events when prepared.

20.1.1.3　Factors that affect stress

(1) The nature of the stressor

From the big side, wars, earthquakes, floods, fires and other disasters will bring heavy psychological pressure and burden to people. From a small aspect, in the face of an examination or assessment, their illness or the illness of relatives and friends will also bring unexpected impact and interference to our normal life, and will also become the source of our psychological pressure. In our life, stress accompanies us like a shadow and has become a part of our life. There is no such thing as a completely stress – free situation. In other words, the absence of pressure is itself a kind of pressure, its name is emptiness.

(2) The number of stressors

Simply put, the more stressful events an individual is exposed to in succession at the same time or over a period of time, the greater the stress, and vice versa.

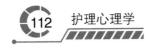

(3) Duration

The longer a stressful event lasts, the more stressful the individual feels, and vice versa.

(4) Predictability

Stress is related to the predictability of stressful events. If individuals can well predict the development direction of stressful events, they may feel less pressure.

(5) Severity

Generally speaking, when the pressure is too high, people's reason is generally difficult to control, individuals often show two extreme behavioral reactions, either numb, completely stop action, or excited, suddenly burst into attack. Moderate psychological stress will generally reduce people's ability to act, repetitive and stereotyped actions. Under moderate pressure or mild pressure, individuals may, under rational control, give full play to the subjective initiative and deal with the pressure events properly, so as to enhance their psychological endurance and increase their dynamic ability.

(6) Coping style

Pressure is a subjective reflection. The magnitude of pressure, namely the intensity of people's psychological feeling of inadaptability, is jointly determined by the objectivity of the stressor event and the subjectivity of self-feeling. Among these two important factors, people's subjective attitude plays a dominant role. Can say the pressure of the size, it is 100% listen to me, I said it is big, it is big; I said it is not big, it is not big; I said no, he did not. Use the formula: pressure = pressure source/bearing capacity.

(7) Social support system

Under pressure, it is best for individuals to rely on their own strength to make light of the clouds. If not, they should actively seek social support and help. When individuals encounter significant pressure and frustration and are difficult to make decisions and bear, we should give priority to the use of counseling help strategy, so that the problem can be properly solved, to establish a network crisis intervention by family, friends, classmates, colleagues. The social support system formed by institutions is an important way to improve the coping ability of stress and frustration

21.1.2 Common stressful events

(1) Pressure from the family: complex family relationships, children's growth problems, marital and romantic relationships, family development problems, major events of family members, etc.

(2) Pressure from the heart: physical needs, security needs, belonging and love needs, respect needs, self-actualization needs, etc.

(3) Pressure from physiology: physical health problems, personal image problems, etc.

(4) Pressure from society: war, natural and man-made disasters, rapid development and changes in society, competition in various industries, handling of interpersonal relationships, setbacks, conflicts, life changes, etc.

Section 2 Response and Harm of Stress

21.2.1 Stress response

21.2.1.1 Physical reactions

When individuals experience stress, the adrenal medulla and adrenal cortex are activated, and the adrenal medulla triggers short-term stress responses and secretes epinephrine and norepinephrine, which eventually leads to a series of physiological reactions, such as elevated blood glucose, constriction of blood vessels, rapid heartbeat, rapid blood diversion from vital organs to the heart and skeletal muscles, resulting in decreased activity of the digestive system, increased metabolic rate of the body, and bronchiectasis. The adrenal cortex triggers a long-term stress response and secretes steroid hormones. Non-corticosteroids trap sodium and water through the kidneys, increasing blood volume and blood pressure, converting protein and fat to glucose or breaking down enzymes, reducing energy and reducing the response of the body's immune system.

21.2.1.2 Psychological reactions

Psychological stress, resulting in a sense of psychological stress, mental tension, difficulty in relaxing, boredom and emptiness, persistent fear or worry, irritability, complaining, self-contradiction, frustration and aggressive tendencies, lack of concentration, slow movement, dejection and anxiety, paranoia, indecision, fear of social difficulties and failure, apathy, world-weariness, lethargy, collapsing, dying, etc.

21.2.1.3 General adaptation syndrome

General adaptation syndrome (GAS), proposed by the Canadian psychologist Hans Selye in the 1930s, believes that this is a type of adaptive response that an individual produces in response to stress: that is, an organism must find its balance or stability in order to maintain or restore its integrity and tranquility, and failure to cope with or adapt to stress may produce "adaptive diseases", namely ulcers, high blood pressure and heart attacks.

General adaptive syndrome consists of 3 phases: alarm, resistance, and depletion.

Phase one, the alarm phase. When the body is exposed to a stressor, it mobilizes energy to meet the demands of the stressor. And show a series of specific changes in the body, such as rapid heartbeat, rapid breathing, a cold sweat. This shows that your body is ready to act immediately. You are ready to masturbate or run away, but if the stimulation is too strong, the body may die

The second stage, the resistance stage. If the stressor has not been eliminated for a long time. Organisms have to face the existence of stressors for a long time. In this case, in order to maintain the internal balance, the organism needs to change to another more complicated state and level to adapt to the stimulus. This response causes the body's various organs and glands to produce various hormones, salts, and sugars to give the energy needed to resist stimuli and maintain the body's internal balance. At this time, the specific index of alert response will disappear, and the various reactions of the organism will exceed the normal level.

The third stage is depletion. After long periods of exposure to the same stressors, the body adapts and the energy it needs to adapt runs out. The characteristic indicators of alert response reappear. The current state is impossible to reverse. When the body can no longer resist pressure in. When the stressors are placed on them, they collapse, collapse, and eventually cause the body to die (Figure 21-1).

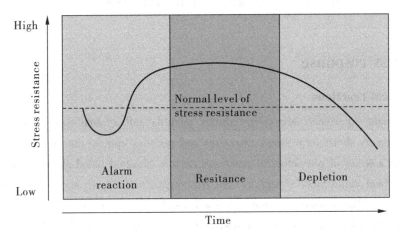

Figure 21-1   Time stages of general adaptation syndrome

21.2.2 Harm of stress to the human body

21.2.2.1 Physiological symptoms

When a person is under too much pressure, the most obvious reaction is muscle tension, rapid heartbeat, increased blood pressure, sweating and other symptoms. Medical scientists have found that when the human body is too stressed, it will seriously affect the health of the human body's nerves, bones, breathing, cardiovascular endocrinology, gastrointestinal, reproduction and other seven major systems. At the same time, high stress can also cause allergies, headaches, eczema, heart disease and other diseases.

21.2.2.2 Psychological symptoms

Excessive stress will cause inattention, memory decline, comprehension, creativity decline; often worried, irritable, anxious. Even neurotic psychological disorders, serious and even emotional indifference, delusions, hallucinations, suicidal ideation and other pathological psychological phenomena.

21.2.2.3 Emotional symptoms

Excessive pressure makes people unhappy, depressed, anxious, painful, dissatisfied, pessimistic and sullen, allergic feelings, feel that life is not interesting, self-control declines, sudden anger, tears or laughter, and the ability to work independently declines. Besides, stress is also easy to make people forgetful, burnout, and less efficient. In addition, people who are too psychologically stressed will become cold and rash.

21.2.2.4 Behavioral symptoms

Excessive stress makes people have negative slacking off, decreased work efficiency, and evasive responses. Excessive pressure is easy to cause people to clash with others, and interpersonal relationships deteriorate. Excessive stress makes people change their habits, such as smoking, alcoholism, and even drug abuse to numb themselves. Even more, they show destructive pathological reactions such as suicide and homicide.

In short, the right amount of pressure over a short period of time can boost productivity and promote change. Long – term stress can lead to changes in people's emotions and behaviors, and even physical illness.

Section 3   Stress Management of Nurses

21.3.1   Main source of nurses' stress

21.3.1.1   Care for the sick

The pressure caused by the heavy nursing work to the nurses, most of the patients lack of disease knowledge, high expectations of medical technical services, think that as long as into the hospital, there is no problem can not be solved, nurses should be submissive to the patients, treatment and nursing operation on slowly, a needle of blood, injections hurt, call for help, do not pay attention to, such as sound not in time will result in the patient's are not satisfied, to nurse a shortfuse, complaints, threats, even make nurses feel work is too passive, wind up everywhere, largely hit the nurses' working enthusiasm, caused a lot of pressure.

21.3.1.2   Stress in the work environment

Hospital nursing work is ordinary, trivial (such as lights are not bright, heating is not hot, air conditioning is not cool, the patient's knife pain, ward accompany more affect the patient's rest, can't find a doctor, they will first look for the nurse to say difficult to listen). The sense of urgency of competition and "three shifts" disrupted the rhythm of life of nurses. In the medical and health system, nurses work the hardest, but their pay is relatively low, and their labor is not rewarded accordingly. When nurses do all kinds of treatment and nursing work, they work under the supervision of patients, family members and even the news media, which increases the psychological pressure of nurses imperceptibly and easily leads to psychosomatic diseases. In addition, nurses are also faced with certain occupational hazards, such as blood-borne infectious diseases, AIDS, syphilis, hepatitis B.

21.3.1.3   Stress outside of work

Nurse is the main composition of the female, as an ordinary working women, in addition to professional responsibility, family responsibility and social responsibility, should be a good doctor's assistant, leadership and patient good nurses, and to do filial daughter and daughter – in – law, loving mother, good wife, work, social and family must balance, therefore, at the same time to undertake a variety of roles. They are increased pressure on nurses.

21.3.1.4   Limited self–development

With the development of modern nursing discipline, the scope of nursing work continues to expand, nurses are required not only to have a high sense of responsibility, good professional ethics, strong clinical skills and keen observation, but also have good communication skills and social adaptability. Professional development, the knowledge structure of updates, various modern rescue technology, the application of advanced instruments, make nurse requirements constantly improve themselves, but the nurse continues to pursue advanced studies and less chance of promotion, there are quite a number of nurses working lifetime learning are not out of the hospital, can't keep pace with the times of mastering new

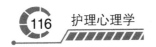

knowledge, new technology and the pressure.

21.3.2　Stress management methods

(1) Develop the ability to adapt and cope with problems. For example, problem – solving techniques, critical thinking. Recognize the nature of stressful events, rationally think and analyze the context of the problem events, and confirm the ability of individuals to deal with problems. Use problem solving skills, develop a solution plan, and actively deal with problems.

(2) Learn relaxation techniques.

1) Breathing exercise: through deep and long inhalation and exhalation, to achieve the effect of relaxation, generally abdominal breathing is the best, that is, the abdomen protrudes during inspiration, and the abdomen is concave when exhaling.

2) Self – generated training: basically, it is a series of spoken formulas for the recipient to repeat to himself or herself, so that he or she can enter a relaxed state. For example, I feel very calm, very easy, my feet feel heavy and loose, and my hands feel heavy and warm.

3) Qigong.

(3) Use your defense mechanisms. The psychological defense mechanism is a natural psychological defense function for people to resist pressure, eliminate bad emotions and get psychological balance when they encounter setbacks. The premise of starting the psychological defense mechanism is to encounter setbacks and stress response. Common are denial, humor, replacement, rationalization, sublimation. Psychological defense mechanisms can help a person avoid or reduce anxiety in a variety of ways, give the other person time to solve problems that might overwhelm him, and help individuals learn new ways to adapt to their environment. But psychological defense mechanisms can only change the way a person thinks and responds to stress, not the stressful situation.

(4) Develop good living habits. Include healthy eating habits, adequate sleep, moderate exercise, reasonable rest.

(5) Make rational decisions, think calmly and rationally in the face of pressure, and effectively control emotions.

(6) Plan your time properly, manage your time well, and prioritize.

(7) Establish a positive and correct outlook on life, avoid overemphasizing work or study, balance all aspects of life, and be good at thinking.

(8) Improve the social support system, be able to honestly share your problems and emotions with family and friends, and also be able to give good empathy to others.

第一章　护理心理学概述

======== **学习目标** ========

1. 掌握心理学、护理心理学的概念。
2. 熟悉护理心理学的研究任务。
3. 了解心理学的相关理论。

第一节　护理心理学简介

一、心理学的概念

心理学(psychology)一词来源于希腊词"psyche",意为"心""心灵";"logos",意为"知识""观念"。心理学是研究人类行为、思维过程和情感的学科。行为是有机体适应环境的方式,分为两类,外显行为和内隐性行为。外显行为是指直接可观察到的行为和反应,如吃、说话。内隐性行为是指内部活动,如思考、做梦和记忆。心理过程或认知过程,指的是我们了解周围世界的所有方式。情感过程是指人对客观事物的态度体验及相应的行为反应。

心理学家从事基础研究的目的是描述、解释、预测和控制行为,从事应用心理学研究的目的是提高人类生活质量。

二、护理心理学的概念

护理心理学是研究如何运用心理学理论、技术和方法,来解决护理实践中的心理问题,以达到最佳的护理效果的一门应用学科。它是心理学与护理学相结合而形成的一门交叉学科。

三、护理心理学的意义

1. 全面提高护理质量　护理的对象是人,人是有复杂心理活动的,护士必须了解人的心理活动,才能使服务对象满意。护士通过学习护理心理学,掌握了患者的心理活动规律,全面地认识了疾病和患者,才有可能采取相应的心理护理技术进行心理护理,这样的护理才会使患者感到生理上舒适、心理上舒畅。患者的这种良好心理状态能够促进其良好的生理功能,良好生理功能又会反过来促进其形成良好的、积极的心理状态。生理与心理的这种积极的交互作用促进病程向健康方向发展,从而全面有效地提高护理质量。

2.培养护士良好心理素质　新的护理环境要求护士应具备良好的心理素质、敏捷的思维、丰富的想象力、精确的语言表达能力、适度的情绪感染力以及良好的沟通能力等。然而,护士也是普通人,各有其气质特点和性格特征,同样受其自身生理、心理、社会变化的影响,可能出现各种情绪和心理的变化,如心理状态调整不好,在一定程度上会对护理工作及其质量带来负面影响。所以,护士应有意识地调节自我心理状态,培养和优化自己的职业心理素质,在护理心理学的理论指导下,在实践中不断强化专业学习,努力使自己成为业务技术精湛、知识结构完善和心理素质优良的护理工作者。

四、护理心理学的研究任务

护理心理学作为一门刚刚兴起的独立学科,理论体系框架还不完善。为了适应现代社会发展的需要,研究者要努力完善其理论体系,不断探索科学应用模式,以此来指导护理实践及临床工作。因此护理心理学的研究任务就显得尤为重要,主要包括以下几个任务。

1.研究护理对象在护理实践中心理变化的规律和特点　个体的先天遗传和后天环境不同,形成的个性心理是不同的。因此,在护理实践中护理对象所表现的心理反应存在很大差异。一般而言,无论患者得了什么病,均会对患者的心理活动产生一定的负面影响,特别是患有一些急性的、严重的、难以治愈和预后不良的疾病更是如此。但不同的护理对象,因个性心理的差异所产生的心理变化和心理反应是不同的。如当知道自己身患癌症时,内向性格的人常会表现出以抑郁为主的急性心理反应;外向性格的人则表现出以愤怒为主的急性心理反应。因此,研究护理对象的个性心理,有利于提高心理护理的成效。

2.研究护理人员在护理实践中的心理变化　护理实践是护理人员与护理对象之间进行的一种互动过程。护理人员具有高尚的职业道德是进行心理护理的前提,具有良好的心理品质是进行心理护理的基础,具有健全的个性心理是进行心理护理的保证,具有娴熟的护理技术是进行心理护理的条件。因此,护理人员的个性心理特征和护理实践时的心理变化都会影响心理护理的成效。

3.研究心理护理的方法　护理是以护理程序为框架针对心理问题开展的系统化护理,分为心理社会评估、心理问题诊断、心理护理计划、心理护理实施和心理护理评价5个步骤。为更好地依照护理的程序进行心理护理,应在良好的护患关系基础上,熟练掌握观察技术、沟通技术、咨询技术、心理评估和干预技术等。敏锐的观察能更准地发现护理对象的心理问题;恰当的沟通既能更多、更快地了解护理对象,又能融洽护患关系;真诚的咨询既有利于改变护理对象错误的护理认知模式,又有利于激发其战胜疾病的信心;准确的心理评估既能对心理问题进行定性和定量评估,为心理护理诊断提供依据,又能为护理科研提供客观资料;精湛的干预技术有助于心理问题的解决。

4.研究和应用心理健康教育的内容与方法　由于心理健康较生理健康更易受周围环境和人群的影响,同时患者生理、心理方面的状态和变化对其亲属所产生的心理影响常常较生理影响大得多,因此对患者及家属进行适当的心理健康教育是十分必要的。对正常人进行适当的心理健康教育,能帮助人们预防某些心理问题的出现,或一旦出现心理问题能及时进行应对。适当的心理健康教育还能帮助人们正确认识某些疾病,消除由于错误认识带来的心理恐惧等。

第二节　心理学重要的理论

心理学家采用很多不同的方法来试图理解人的心理,不同的方法形成不同的观点。这些观点多年来一直在变化,但最常见的有心理动力学理论、行为主义理论、人本主义理论和认知理论。

一、心理动力学理论

心理动力学理论,又称精神分析理论,在19世纪末由西格蒙德·弗洛伊德(1856—1936)提出,然后由埃里克森、荣格和克莱因发展。精神动力学一个关键的组成部分是激发一个人行为的内在或无意识的冲突,认为童年经历对成人人格的形成至关重要。弗洛伊德把人的心理结构分为意识、潜意识和前意识3个层次,并形象地把其比喻为漂浮在大海上的一座冰山。

1.意识　指个体在觉醒状态下所能感知到的心理部分,能被自我意识所知觉,它只是个体心理活动的有限的外显部分。意识能保持个体对环境和自我状态的感知,对人的适应有重要作用。弗洛伊德曾做过比喻,认为心理活动的意识部分好比海平面以上的冰山的山尖部分,而潜意识则是海洋下面看不到的巨大的冰山部分。

2.潜意识　又称无意识,指个体在觉醒状态下无法直接感知到的心理部分,如已被意识遗忘了的童年不愉快的经历、心理的创伤、无法得到满足的情感经验和本能、欲望与冲动等,潜意识的内容通常不能被外部现实、道德和理智等接受。

3.前意识　介于意识和潜意识之间,指目前不在意识之中,但通过集中注意或提醒能被带到意识层面的心理部分。前意识的作用是对欲望和需求的控制,使其尽可能按照外界现实规范的要求和个人道德来调节,是意识和潜意识之间的缓冲区。

精神分析理论是最早的系统解释人类心理及行为的心理学体系,对理解和解释人类的心理现象及其规律有重要的贡献,也是心理治疗重要的取向,对维护心理健康和预防心理疾病有重要作用。

二、行为主义理论

行为主义理论,又称"刺激-反应-结果"理论,是20世纪20年代美国心理学家华生在俄国心理学家巴甫洛夫(Pavlov)的经典条件反射理论基础上建立的。美国心理学家斯金纳和班杜拉等进一步完善和发展了行为主义理论。

从19世纪末开始,俄国生理学家巴甫洛夫进行了著名的条件反射实验研究。实验的第一步:用食物刺激使狗的口腔产生唾液分泌反应,食物是非条件刺激,所引起唾液分泌的反射过程称为非条件反射。非条件反射是本能行为,是不学自能的。例如婴儿出生后即有吮吸反射和拥抱反射等。实验的第二步:每次给狗食物时,总是配合以铃声出现,即将食物与另一种与唾液分泌原本无关的中性环境刺激例如铃声总是配对出现。实验的第三步:经过一定时间的训练,单独铃声刺激也会引起狗的唾液分泌。此时,这种中性刺激(铃声)变成了条件刺激。铃声引起唾液分泌的反射过程就是条件反射。通过条件反射习得的行为不能被个体随意操作和控制,属于反应性行为,也称为经典条件反射。

操作条件反射理论强调行为结果对行为本身的作用。该理论是由美国心理学家斯金纳等人通过动物实验建立的。实验在著名的斯金纳箱中进行。饥饿的老鼠在实验箱中会出现一系列的盲目行为,如乱叫、乱咬、乱窜、按压杠杆等,只有按压杠杆后,老鼠才能获得食物,即"食物的出现"对"按压杠杆"的动作起到了促进和加强的效果。经过多次实验,老鼠就学会了按压杠杆获取食物的行为,即在操作杠杆和获取食物之间建立了条件反射。像这种伴随着行为(操作杠杆)出现的结果(食物出现)对行为本身产生的加强效果称为强化,刺激结果称为强化物。同样,在回避操作条件实验中,动物受到电击会产生一系列的行为反应(如乱叫、乱咬、乱窜、回避等),其中的一种行为反应,即回避动作出现时,即可获得撤销电击的结果。撤销电击的结果对回避行为有加强效果,结果动物学会了回避行为。以上实验说明,当某一行为(如按压杠杆行为或回避行为)出现时总能获得某种积极的结果(食物出现或撤销电击),则个体逐渐学会对这种行为的操作,这就是操作条件反射。

社会观察学习(social learning)理论的代表人物是班杜拉,强调人的社会行为是通过观察学习获得的,并没有得到直接的强化和奖励,个体仅仅通过观察他人的行为反应就可达到模仿学习的目的。在护理工作中,该理论有重要的应用价值。例如,患者角色行为的形成与示范作用有一定关系,包括喊叫、呻吟及应对方式等;同样,示范作用原则也可用于对患者的指导和护理,以及儿童患者的教育等。

三、人本主义理论

人本主义理论,20 世纪五六十年代兴起于美国,代表人物是马斯洛和罗杰斯,重视人的尊严、价值、创造力和自我实现,强调人是具有潜能的个体,自我实现归结为潜能的发挥。

人本主义理论的贡献是强调个体在心理发展中的重要作用,是让个体领悟到自己的本性,由自己的意志来决定自己的行为,修复被破坏的自我实现潜力,促进个体的健康发展。在此基础上发展的来访者中心疗法,也是目前心理咨询与治疗中的主导疗法之一。

四、认知理论

认知理论起源于 20 世纪 50 年代,与认知心理学发展密切相关。认知心理学主要研究人类认识的信息加工过程,并以此来解释人类的复杂行为,如概念的形成、问题的解决、语言及情感等。认知理论认为,认知对情绪和行为具有决定作用,思想和信念是情绪状态和行为表现的原因。在此基础上美国心理学家埃利斯和贝克分别提出了情绪的 ABC 理论和情绪障碍认知理论,并发展了相应的认知治疗的理论和技术。

练习题

1. 研究如何运用心理学理论、技术和方法,来解决护理实践中的心理问题,以达到最佳的护理效果的一门应用学科是(　　)
    A. 普通心理学　　　　B. 应用心理学　　　　C. 医学心理学　　　　D. 护理心理学
2. 新的护理环境要求护士应具备的能力不包括(　　)
    A. 良好的心理素质　　B. 敏捷的思维　　　　C. 较深的文字写作能力　D. 适度的情绪感染力
3. 心理动力学理论,又称(　　)
    A. 精神分析理论　　　B. 人本主义理论　　　C. 心理发展理论　　　D. 行为主义理论
4. 心理动力学理论的创立者是(　　)
    A. 埃里克森　　　　　B. 西格蒙德·弗洛伊德　C. 荣格　　　　　　　D. 克莱因

5.弗洛伊德把人的心理结构分为 3 个层次,不包括( )

　　A.意识　　　　　　　B.潜意识　　　　　　C.前意识　　　　　　D.有意识

6.行为主义理论是创立者是( )

　　A.华生　　　　　　　B.巴甫洛夫　　　　　C.斯金纳　　　　　　D.班杜拉

7.巴甫洛夫进行了著名的条件反射实验研究中铃声引起唾液分泌属于( )

　　A.条件刺激　　　　　B.条件反射　　　　　C.非条件刺激　　　　D.非条件反射

8.操作条件反射理论提出者是( )

　　A.班杜拉　　　　　　B.斯金纳　　　　　　C.巴甫洛夫　　　　　D.罗杰斯

9.下列关于人本主义理论观点说法错误的是( )

　　A.重视人的尊严、价值、创造力和自我实现　　B.强调人是具有潜能的个体

　　C.强调人的社会行为是通过观察学习获得的　　D.自我实现归结为潜能的发挥

10.认知理论的观点认为( )

　　A.认知对情绪和行为具有决定作用

　　B.强调人是具有潜能的个体

　　C.个体仅仅通过观察他人的行为反应就可达到模仿学习的目的

　　D.认为童年经历对成人人格的形成至关重要

参考答案

第二章　发展心理学概述

1. 掌握影响成长和发展的因素。
2. 熟悉人类发展的领域和发展的原则。
3. 了解人类的成长和发展的概念。

第一节　发展心理学研究概述

一、成长

成长,一般指个体长大、长成成人,也泛指事物走向成熟,摆脱稚嫩的过程。简单概括来讲,就是自身不断变得成熟稳重的变化过程。成长是向一个方向靠近,这个方向是个体所在社会人际圈的特定强权所有者的特定年龄。一般来讲,我们对于成长的解释就是个体身体和心理向成熟发展的经历。

二、发展

发展指事物由小到大,由简到繁,由低级到高级,由旧物质到新物质的运动变化过程。心理学认为人的发展是指从出生到死亡在身心方面所发生的所有规律的变化过程,是一个从多级量变到质变的过程。它包括了生理发展和心理发展两个方面。①生理发展:是指机体的各种组织系统(骨骼、肌肉、心脏、神经系统、呼吸系统等)的发育及其功能的增长,即指功能的正常发育和体质的增强。②心理发展:指个体有规律的心理变化,包括知识的发展、智力的发展和意向的发展。

三、个体发展阶段

第一个阶段:受孕到出生。这个阶段也称为产前时期,从一个受精卵发育成胚胎,再到胎儿,最后新生儿诞生。

第二个阶段:出生到1岁。这个阶段也称为婴儿期或者新生儿期。这个阶段认为是所有阶段中最重要的阶段,最不能被忽视的阶段,这阶段的重点是孩子与母亲和其他主要抚养人之间建立良好的依恋关系。父母对孩子的抚养方式、对孩子的态度,应该是建立在一种规律性的基础之上,不能使孩子经常体验到一种不确定性。同时这个时期,婴儿自己,对人生是乐观的、自信的、勇敢的,有强烈的探索这个世界和自我实现的欲望。

第三个阶段:1~6岁。这个时期是孩子的孩提时代。主要是儿童的自主性、独立性发展,和学习遵守生活规则、社会规范。在这个年段,孩子的认知能力开始发展,孩子的自我意识开始形成,孩子处于第一反抗期。自主性、独立性的发展对孩子的一生都非常重要,但是孩子也要学习去遵守生活规范与社会规则。这常常使很多父母在这两个问题上左右摇摆,对孩子的管教究竟是松一些,还是严一些,父母们常常不知道如何去处理。在这个阶段主要是发展孩子的想象力和创造力。

第四个阶段:6~12岁,也称为童年时期。这阶段主要是形成孩子的勤奋感和责任心。我们知道这两种品质对一生是非常重要。如果孩子具有这两种品质,父母就不需要为孩子的一生担忧。我们说穷人的孩子早当家。这些孩子很小就知道对自己、他人负责任,很勤奋地去学习、劳动。此期孩子已具备了足够的自给自足和自我保护的能力和智慧,并且在循序渐进地摆脱父母和社会对自己的干预和影响,寻求自我的独立和开放,敢于做真实的、与生俱来的、纯真的自己。这时候,孩子会变得越来越自信、勇敢和有担当。

第五个阶段:13岁左右到成人,就是我们讲的青春期。埃里克森认为是角色认同的阶段、同一性的阶段。即是孩子迈向成人的最后阶段,是为成人做好所有准备的阶段,也是现在全世界工业化社会中最为感到迷惘、头痛的阶段。心理问题的产生,往往是因为当事人固结在了童年时期,还是感觉自己很弱小,不具备自给自足、自我保护的能力和智慧,继续采用原来的策略寻求给养和保护。所表现出来的就是自卑、胆怯、不敢承担责任。具体的心理问题是焦虑、恐惧、强迫、抑郁和矛盾、冲突。

第六个阶段:成年期,即25~60岁这个年龄段。按成年人的心理和生理特点,又可分为3个阶段:青年晚期(25~30岁),成年前期(30~40岁),成年中期(40~60岁)。在成年期,人的身体发育成熟,各种生理活动相对稳定。就脑的发展而言,20岁以前脑的成熟过程已基本完成,但某些方面还在发展着。髓鞘化过程是脑发展的一个重要指标,网状组织的髓鞘化过程延续到30多岁。作为智力过程的生理基础的大脑联合区一直发展到老年。但随着年龄的增长,人体各器官系统的功能开始向衰退过渡。特别是在成年中期以后,身体各种功能,如体力、精力、抵抗力呈下降趋势并随年龄的增加而日渐明显。所以,青年晚期和成年前期是人生的黄金时期,体力、精力旺盛,社会经验和文化知识丰富,成为社会各项事业、生产和活动的基本力量,是家庭养老、育儿的主要承担者,一定要珍惜这段时期。

最后一个阶段:衰老。从生物学上讲,衰老是生物随着时间的推移,自发的必然过程,它是复杂的自然现象,表现为结构的退行性变和功能的衰退,适应性和抵抗力减退。在生理学上,把衰老看作是从受精卵开始一直到老年的个体发育史。从病理学上,衰老是应激和劳损、损伤和感染、免疫反应衰退、营养失调、代谢障碍以及疏忽和滥用药物积累的结果。另外从社会学上看,衰老是个人对新鲜事物失去兴趣,超脱现实,喜欢怀旧的过程。衰老是没有明确的界限,同时也是不可避免的,主要是以生理和心理的变化为标准。

第二节　个体成长和发展的原则及其影响因素

一、发展的原则

孩子在生长发育过程中遵循一定的规则。

1. 先头后脚原则　指从上到下的发展顺序,儿童身体的发展严格地遵循着头颈—躯干—下肢的次序进行。先发展头部和上半身的能力,再发展身体的其他部分。

2. 由近及远原则　指从中轴向外围的发展顺序,儿童运动的发展顺序是从躯干开始向四肢再向手和脚,最后达到手指和脚趾的小肌肉运动。近,指的是近心脏。先发展躯干再发展四肢功能。孩子学习使用自己身体的各个部分,也遵循这个原则。比如,先学会挥动手臂,再学会使用手指。

3. 从简单到复杂原则　先独立发展简单的技能,再把各种简单的技能整合起来,形成更加复杂的技能。比如,先学会抓勺子,再学会用勺子把食物放进嘴里。后者除了简单的抓握技能,还需要手眼协调配合。

4. 系统独立性原则　人体的不同系统按不同的发展速率各自发展。比如,骨骼肌肉、神经系统、性器官都分属不同的系统,发展模式各不相同。

二、影响个体发展的因素

1. 遗传影响　遗传是一种生理现象,是指双亲的身体结构和功能的各种特征通过遗传基因传递给下一代的现象。遗传的生物特征,或称遗传素质,主要是指那些与生俱来的有机体的构造、形态、感官和神经系统等方面的解剖生理特征。生理成熟是指机体生长发育的程度或水平,也称为生理发展。

2. 环境影响　环境使遗传所提供的心理发展的可能性变为现实,尽管遗传提供了心理发展的可能性,但如果不生活在社会环境里,这种可能性也不会变成现实。野兽抚养大的孩子虽然具有人类的遗传素质,却不具备人类的正常心理。环境是指围绕在个体周围的并对个体自发地产生潜移默化作用的外部世界。即围绕在个体周围的自然环境和社会环境。这里不包括有目的地对人施加影响的教育活动。主要是指家庭所处的地理环境、文化传统、风俗习惯、政治背景、社会关系以及社会风气等。这些都影响着一个人的发展。

三、影响个体生长发育的因素

1. 营养　合理的营养是小儿生长发育的物质基础,年龄越小受营养的影响越大。宫内营养不良的胎儿,不仅体格生长落后,脑的发育也迟缓;生后长期营养不良首先导致体重不增,最终也会影响身高的增长和使机体的免疫、内分泌、神经调节等功能低下,影响智力、心理和社会适应能力的发展。儿童摄入过多热量所致的肥胖也会对其生长发育造成严重影响。

2. 疾病和药物　疾病对小儿生长发育的影响十分明显。急性感染常使体重减轻,长期慢性疾病则同时影响体重和身高的增长;内分泌疾病常引起骨骼生长和神经系统发育迟缓;先天性疾病如先天性心脏病、21-三体综合征等,对体格和神经心理发育的影响更为明显。有些药物也可影响小儿的生长发育,如较大剂量或较长时间给予链霉素、庆大霉素可致听力减退,甚至耳聋;长期应用肾上腺糖皮质激素可致身高增长的速度减慢。

　　3.孕母情况　胎儿在宫内的发育受孕母生活环境、营养、情绪、健康状况等因素的影响。如妊娠早期感染风疹、带状疱疹、巨细胞病毒,可导致胎儿先天畸形;孕母患严重营养不良可引起流产、早产和胎儿体格生长以及脑的发育迟缓;孕母接受药物、放射线、其他环境污染和精神创伤等,均可使胎儿发育受阻。宫内发育阻滞可影响小儿出生后的生长发育。另外,孕妇可以把她所想所闻,甚至梦中的感觉,转变成胎内环境的变化信息,在不知不觉中传给胎儿。胎儿生长发育所需要的营养,是由孕妇通过胎盘提供的。孕妇不良的情绪变化会影响营养的摄取、激素的分泌和血液的生化成分,以致血液中有害于神经系统和其他组织器官的物质激增,并通过胎盘影响胎儿发育,进而导致胎儿畸形。

练习题

1.发展心理学的研究对象是(　　　)

　　A.个体从出生到衰亡全过程的心理发展现象　　B.解释心理发展现象

　　C.揭示心理发展规律　　　　　　　　　　　　D.描述心理发展现象、揭示心理发展规律

2.发展心理学研究的是(　　　)

　　A.认知发展规律　　　B.心理的种族发展　　C.心理的种系发展　　D.心理发展规律

3.以下不属于影响个体身体和心理发展的因素是(　　　)

　　A.遗传　　　　　　　B.环境　　　　　　　C.母体　　　　　　　D.性别

4.以下不属于个体心理发展的特点是(　　　)

　　A.从简单到复杂　　　B.从高级到低级　　　C.从无到有　　　　　D.单一到完善

参考答案

第三章 婴儿的发展

第一节 婴儿的生理发展

婴儿生理发展是指其大脑和身体在形态、结构及功能上的生长发育过程。大脑、神经系统和感官的活动是心理活动的基础。婴儿的生理发展直接影响并制约着婴儿心理的发生发展过程,因此婴儿生理的发展一直是研究的重要课题。

一、婴儿的身体发展

(一)婴儿大脑的形态发展

1. 脑重与头围　婴儿大脑从胚胎时期开始发育,出生时重量为 350～400 g,是成人脑重的 25%。此后第一年内脑重增长最快,6 个月为 700～800 g,12 个月为 800～900 g。这些发展变化在一定程度上反映了各个阶段大脑内部结构发育和成熟的情况,与大脑皮质面积的发展密切相关。同时,婴儿头围也存在类似的发展变化。刚出生时头围已达 34 cm 左右,12 个月时达 46～47 cm。

2. 大脑皮质　胎儿六七个月时,脑基本结构就已具备。出生时脑细胞已分化,细胞结构筑区和层次分化已基本上完成,大多数沟回已出现,岛叶已被邻近脑叶掩盖,脑内基本感觉运动通路已髓鞘化(白质除外)。此后,婴儿皮质细胞迅速发展,层次拓展,神经元密度下降且相互分化,突触装置日趋复杂化。

(二)婴儿大脑的功能发展

1. 脑电活动　脑电活动的变化常常作为婴儿脑发展的一个重要指标。研究证实,5 个月的胎儿已显示出脑电活动,8 个月以后则呈现出与新生儿相同的脑电图,脑电活动开始具有连续性和初步的节律性,形成睡眠和觉醒的脑电图。出生后 5 个月是婴儿脑电活动发展的重要阶段。脑电逐渐皮质化,伴随着产生皮质下抑制。5～12 个月,外部刺激引起的诱发电位发生变化,如视觉诱发电位构型变得复杂化,潜伏期缩短等。

2. 皮质中枢　婴儿大脑是按照其基因结构的顺序而发展,遵循着头尾原则和远近原则。婴儿刚出生时大脑两半球及其皮质尚不能正常发挥功能,皮质兴奋还处于弥漫状态,因而只要触动新生儿身体任何部位都会引起其头、手和足等的乱动。

(三)婴儿身体发展过程及其正常值

婴儿身体发展过程指身体各部及各种器官、组织的结构和功能生长发育的过程。生长指量的增加,如身长、体重和各器官的增长;发育是指质的变化,如各器官、组织结构和功能的不断分化、成熟等。

1.体重　刚出生时,足月男婴体重为 3.3~3.4 kg,足月女婴体重为 3.2~3.3 kg。在正常喂养下,到 5 个月婴儿体重增加 1 倍,12 个月时增加 2 倍。

2.身高　刚出生时,足月新生儿身高约为 50 cm。其中,男婴比女婴略高,头胎比第二、三胎略矮。同时受婴儿出生时的体形和营养影响,第一年每月增长约 2.54 cm。

3.头围　刚出生时头围已达 34 cm 左右,0~3 个月时,每月增长 2 cm;4~6 个月时,每月增长 1 cm;6~12 个月时,每月增长 0.5 cm;1~2 岁时,一年增长 2 cm。

4.牙齿　婴儿的牙齿,根据其位置、形态和功能,可分为切牙、犬牙和乳磨牙。婴儿的乳牙在出生后 6~9 个月开始生长。

二、婴儿的动作发展

婴儿各种运动、动作的发展是其活动发展的直接前提,也是其心理发展的外在表现。婴儿动作发展有严密、细致的内在规律,遵循一定的原则,是一个复杂多变而又有规律可循的动态发展系统。

一般认为,婴儿动作最早发生在新生儿期,其最初的非条件反射行为便是"最早产生"的动作。早期人类反射指没有经过学习,在某些刺激出现的时候自动产生的有组织的自然反应。吮吸反射和吞咽反射:进食;定向反射:找到乳头;咳嗽、打喷嚏、眨眼。婴儿对于自己肌肉的控制能力不断增强,部分反射会逐渐消失,成为日后掌握更加复杂行为的基础,帮助复杂行为的发生发展。

第二节　婴儿的认知发展

一、感知觉发展

在婴儿的认知能力中,感知觉是最先发展且发展速度最快的一个领域,在婴儿认知活动中一直占主导地位。

1.视觉的发生发展　目前大量研究已经证实,视觉最初发生的时间是在胎儿中晚期,即 4~5 个月的胎儿已有了视觉反应能力以及相应的生理基础。新生儿已具备一定的视觉能力,获得了基本的视觉过程,并具备了原始的颜色视觉。2~4 个月婴儿的颜色知觉已发展得很好。另外,大量研究证实婴儿至少在 6 个月已确实具有了明显的立体觉。

2.听觉的发生发展　近年来,越来越多的心理学家认为,正常健康婴儿一生下来就有听觉,听觉可以说是与生俱来的。目前关于婴儿研究的最新成果表明,5~6 个月胎儿已开始建立听觉系统,可以听到透过母体的 1 000 Hz 以下的声音。对于听敏度的发展,1 个月婴儿能鉴别 200 Hz 与 500 Hz纯音之间的差异。5~8 个月婴儿可在 1 000~3 000 Hz 范围觉察出声频的 2% 的变化,在 4 000~8 000 Hz的差别阈限与成人水平相同。

视听协调能力的发展:刚出生的婴儿就有最基本的视听协调能力。3~6个月婴儿的视听协调能力已发展到能使他判别视听信息是否一致的水平。

3.味觉、嗅觉和触觉的发生发展 在婴儿4个月时已经能感受到足够的味觉刺激,新生儿的味觉发育得相当完好,在其防御反射机制中占有相当重要的地位。味觉在婴儿和儿童时期最发达,以后逐渐衰退。婴儿7~8个月时嗅觉感受器已相当成熟且具有了初步的嗅觉反应能力,已能大致区别几种不同的气味。新生儿已能对各种气味作出相应的典型反应,如"喜爱"好闻的气味等。还能由嗅觉建立食物性条件反射,并有初步的嗅觉空间定位能力。对于触觉,婴儿在第49天就已经具有初步的触觉反应,2个月时能对细而尖的刺激产生反应活动。新生儿能够凭口腔触觉分辨软硬不同的乳头,4个月时则能同时分辨不同形状和软硬程度的乳头。本能性触觉反应在婴儿刚出生时便可表现出来,4个月以后的婴儿则具有成熟的够物行为,视触协调能力已发展起来。

二、注意的发生发展

婴儿一生下来就有注意。这种注意实质上就是先天的定向反射,是无意注意的最初形态。新生儿已有了注意的选择性,并具备了对外界进行扫视的能力。1~3个月的婴儿的注意已经明显地偏向曲线、不规则图形或复杂刺激物。3~6个月婴儿平均注意时间缩短,偏爱更加复杂和有意义的视觉对象。6个月以后婴儿的睡眠时间减少,注意不再像以前那样只表现在视觉等方面,而是以更广泛和更复杂的形成表现在吮吸、抓握等日常活动中。

第三节 婴儿情绪、社会性发展

一、情绪发展

从出生起,婴儿就是一个社会的人,婴儿就被包围在各种社会物体、社会刺激之中,形成和发展着人的情绪情感、社会行为和关系等。

儿童出生后就有情绪表现,如新生儿哭、静、四肢蹬动。同时,初生婴儿的情绪反应及已经初步分化。情绪专家伊扎德研究表明,人类婴儿在出生时,就展示出了5种不同的情绪,分别是惊奇、伤心、厌恶、高兴和兴趣。我国心理学家孟昭兰研究表明,新生儿具有好奇、厌恶、痛苦和微笑4种表情。可见,婴儿出生后不仅有情绪,而且已经初步分化。

二、婴儿情绪的社会化

初生婴儿的情绪都是生理性的,是一种原始本能的反应,由机体内外某些适宜、不适宜的刺激所引起,并反映机体当时的内部状态、生理需要。婴儿社会性微笑、陌生人焦虑、分离焦虑和情绪的社会性参照等是婴儿情绪社会化的核心内容。

第四节 婴儿的护理

作为一名护士,与婴儿建立信任很重要。按照埃里克森人格发展理论,婴儿期处在基本信任与不信任的冲突时期。此时若认为婴儿是一个不懂事的小动物,只要吃饱不哭就行,那就大错特错了。此时是基本信任和不信任的心理冲突期,因为这期间孩子开始认识人了,当孩子哭或饿时,父母是否出现则是建立信任感的重要问题。信任在人格中形成了"希望"这一品质,它起着增强自我的力量。具有信任感的儿童敢于希望,富于理想,具有强烈的未来定向。反之则不敢希望,时时担忧自己的需要得不到满足。埃里克森把希望定义为:"对自己愿望的可实现性的持久信念,反抗黑暗势力、标志生命诞生的怒吼。"

因此在这个阶段对婴儿的护理包括以下这几种方式。

1.满足吸吮需求 通过吸吮宝宝不仅可以得到食物,更能获得安全感。在宝宝出生后到1岁期间,如果父母发现宝宝有这方面的需求,可利用安抚奶嘴来满足。等到宝宝会走路之后,环境中的许多新奇事物会转移他对奶嘴的注意力,所以无须过分担心戒不掉奶嘴的问题。由于探索需求旺盛,凡是能拿到的东西,1岁半以内的宝宝都喜欢往嘴巴里塞,有时不免让父母感到紧张。其实,当宝宝的嘴巴接触到不同软硬、大小及触感的东西时,更能刺激他的感官能力的发展,所以一般不要禁止婴儿吮吸的需要。

2.建立饮食习惯 在宝宝开始长牙之后,就要训练吃辅食,辅食的咀嚼过程也是在满足宝宝的口腔需求。这时需要培养宝宝良好的饮食习惯,包括固定的用餐时间、不偏食、愿意尝试不同口感的食物、专心进食等。由于咀嚼是口腔期宝宝满足需求的方式之一,所以吃辅食能协助宝宝顺利过渡到固体食物阶段,会转移他对乳头、奶嘴及奶瓶的需求,也就不会出现对奶嘴过度依赖而戒不掉的情况。

3.不要吝惜对婴儿的拥抱 许多人认为宝宝一哭就抱并不好,这样容易养成婴儿过分依赖的个性,其实并不是这样。请不要吝惜拥抱宝宝,当他真的需要拥抱时,父母的拥抱与安抚不但给宝宝带来温暖的关爱,更能增进他对世界的信赖,消除心中的不安全感,对于孩子一生的发展都极为有益。

同时,也要对不同的婴幼儿采取不同的心理护理。有些孩子安静容易满足;有些则需要更多的疼爱和关爱,因此看护者应充满爱心、自信,镇定、有耐心地多与孩子沟通,使其具有安全感,更快地安定下来。

练习题

1.下列哪项不是婴儿动作发展遵循的原则(　　　)

　　A.顺序原则　　　　　　　B.大小原则　　　　　　C.近远原则　　　　　　D.头尾原则

2.婴儿期常常出现的"破涕为笑"反映了情绪的(　　　)

　　A.易受感染性　　　　　　B.冲动性　　　　　　　C.两极性　　　　　　　D.不稳定性

3.婴儿感知觉的发展是(　　　)

　　A.被动的过程　　　　　　　　　　　　　　　B.主动的、有选择性的心理过程

　　C.过程非常缓慢　　　　　　　　　　　　　　D.成熟较晚

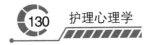

4.新生儿视觉和听觉的集中,是下列哪项发生的标志(　　)

　　A.感觉　　　　　　　　B.知觉　　　　　　　　C.记忆　　　　　　　　D.注意

5.婴儿出生最早表现的特征是(　　)

　　A.能力　　　　　　　　B.个性　　　　　　　　C.性格　　　　　　　　D.气质

参考答案

第四章 幼儿的发展

1. 掌握幼儿护理工作。
2. 熟悉幼儿早期阶段身体、认知、社交和情感发展特点。
3. 了解幼儿发展的心理特征。

第一节 幼儿的生理、认知发展

一、幼儿的生理发展

1～3岁为幼儿期。婴儿期的生长发育速度是人类一生中最快的阶段,1岁以后的幼儿身体生长发育速度开始减慢。但与其他时期相比,增长速度仍然很快。1岁以后,幼儿的智力和活动力都在迅速的发展,主要表现为身体的结构方面发生了许多重要的变化和幼儿的好奇心不断增长,逐渐地发展了独立意识和对环境不断进行探索的需求。

二、幼儿的认知发展

1～3岁这个阶段的儿童处于无条件接受期。这一时期儿童的生活环境主要是家庭,接触最多的是父母。社会对儿童的要求包括基本生活能力、感觉运动能力发展、运用言语能力和交往能力,如辨认物体和人、学习进食、学习控制大小便、用言语表达自己的要求、称呼人、执行一些简单指令。

(一)感知觉能力的发展

感觉能力和知觉能力是两种不同的能力,但又密切相关。感觉是反映当前客观事物的个别属性的认识过程,如物体的声、色、冷、热、软、硬等。幼儿最早出现的是皮肤感觉(触觉、痛觉、温觉),其后逐步表现出敏锐的嗅觉、味觉、视觉和听觉。

知觉是反映当前客观事物整体特性的认识过程,它是在感觉的基础上形成的。任何一个客观事物,都包含多方面的属性,单纯靠某一种感觉是不能把握的。婴儿半岁左右能够坐起来的时候,可以较好地完成眼手协调的活动。在视觉的调节下,手在视野范围内完成操纵、摆弄物品的活动,这是利用知觉能力综合认识物品的特性。一直到3周岁左右,都是各种知觉能力飞快发展的时期。

(二)运动能力提高

儿童在这个时期学会走路,开始说话,出现表象思维和想象等人类所特有的活动。出现独立

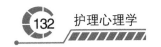

性,各种心理活动逐渐齐全,主要特征为学会直立行走和使用工具。1~3岁儿童学习使用工具有一个过程,大致经过4个阶段。第一阶段,完全不按工具的特点支配动作。第二阶段,不再连续变换新方式,进行同一动作的时间有所延长。第三阶段,主动去重复有效动作。第四阶段,能够按照工具的特点来使用它,并且能够根据使用时的客观条件改变动作方式。2~3岁能够学会多种动作,不仅双手协调,而且能使全身和四肢的动作协调起来。

(三)好奇心旺盛

由于幼儿生性好动,好奇心强,缺少生活经验,综合判断力差,所以特别容易发生意外事故。婴幼儿常见的意外事故有摔倒、误吞异物、烧(烫)伤、触电、煤气中毒、食物中毒和车祸。如有的家长为了不让孩子喝酒或碰其他液体状的东西,而把东西藏起来,但不明确告诉孩子原因,结果孩子很好奇家长到底藏了什么好东西,趁家长不注意就偷喝了,造成食物中毒;有的孩子因为好奇把筷子、牙签等细物往鼻腔、耳腔塞,造成事故时有发生。

第二节　幼儿期情感和人格发展

一、家长情感陪护

与他人的关系对幼儿情感和人格发展至关重要,对幼儿的行为与满足、认可、自我价值和安全感有重要影响。0~3岁是建立情感依赖的关键时期。这个年龄的孩子非常依赖父母,如果长时间变换抚养人,会让孩子很难对别人产生依赖。

这个时期的儿童需要家长的情感陪护。他们更加敏感,因此不应该将教育委托给他人进行。比如孩子长大以后会觉得给父母足够的钱,他们就会快乐,这和家长们在孩子小的时候,对孩子们的爱是一样的。情感抚养期的孩子必须是家长自己进行培养,才可以让长大后的孩子有丰富的情感体验。

二、依恋行为与分离焦虑

3岁幼儿人格发展的另一个重要方面是依恋行为的形成与发展。依恋行为通常指婴幼儿寻找并保持与抚养者(通常是父母)亲密关系的行为倾向和表现。依恋行为的形成与发展对将来的社会化和人际关系发展有重大影响。依恋行为形成和发展是双向的,一方面是婴幼儿寻求保护,对父母的亲昵和依恋行为;另一方面是父母对婴幼儿的关心和依恋,父母的行为同时对婴幼儿产生影响,促进婴幼儿认识世界,形成信赖与不信赖、安全感与不安全感等人格特征。如被隔离抚养的婴幼儿(孤儿院的儿童)由于缺乏与人的交往,依恋行为的形成和发展受到限制,其长大后可出现对人冷漠、孤独,缺乏社会交往等人格特征。

三、幼儿的独立意识

美国心理学家曾对1 500位儿童进行长期追踪观察,30年后发现20%的人没有取得什么成就。与其中成就最大的20%的人对比,发现最显著的差异并不在智力方面,而在于个性品质不同。成就卓越者都是有坚强毅力、独立性和勇往直前等个性品质的人。可见孩子的独立品格对成长和成才是何等重要。

此期人格发展的特点是儿童自我概念初步形成,知道自己与别人的差异,表现出各种基本情绪活动特点,如焦虑、恐惧、羞怯、敌意和愤怒。性格的内向或外向特征也在这一阶段逐渐明显。根据艾里克森的观点,儿童在这一时期面临着信赖危机和自主危机。若儿童在 1 岁左右得到适当照顾,如来自父母温暖、关心和爱,必要的生理和感情需要的满足,则儿童形成信赖感,危机得以解决,产生希望品质,否则出现信赖危机,产生不信任和焦虑感。

第三节 幼儿的健康护理

对幼儿健康护理包括以下 3 点:身体、社会能力和心理护理。从这些方面着手进行护理,更有利于幼儿形成健康的自我意识,培养其独立性,更好地为适应社会生活做准备。

一、身体护理

对幼儿身体护理包括体重、身高、生命体征、视力和听力等。

研究表明,1~3 岁是幼儿大脑飞速发展的关键期,新生儿的脑重约为成人脑重的 25%(350~400 g),1 岁宝宝的脑重量相当于成人的 50%,2 岁宝宝的脑重约为成人的 75%,3 岁宝宝的脑重已经接近成人脑重。这就说明幼儿 3 岁后,智商、体能、性格等方面都已经差不多定型。人类的大脑皮质中存在着 140 亿个神经细胞,也称作"神经元"。神经元之间会形成连接,叫作"神经回路"。神经回路越丰富,大脑就越活跃,行为表现也就越聪明。

如果家长能够在 1~3 岁给幼儿提供的视觉、听觉、触觉、运动和平衡等方面的刺激越多,幼儿大脑的神经回路密度就越高,幼儿就会越聪明。如果缺乏环境刺激,幼儿的大脑发育受到阻碍,大脑重量可减少 20%,且脑神经回路密度也会受到极大程度影响。过了 3 岁关键期,父母很难为幼儿弥补这种损失,也就是说 1~3 岁幼儿的大脑发育是个不可逆的过程。

对于幼儿,必须让其在大脑得到放松后才能正常发育和"消化"所学到的知识。因此新生儿每天的睡眠时间约为 20 h,1 岁后幼儿需要保持 12~15 h。

二、社会能力护理

对于 1~3 岁的幼儿,父母们可以适当地带他们去户外了解外面的世界,如可以带他们去公园里转一转。虽然孩子可能还不太会说话,但是外面事物对幼儿的刺激可以使孩子们的发育得到良好的促进。对于 3~4 岁的孩子,父母可以带其去动物园或海洋馆等场所,这样不仅可以增长他们的知识,而且对于父母与孩子之间良好的亲子感情也起到了促进的作用。此外,也可以带孩子去了解公益,让孩子了解奉献精神,这样不仅可以丰富孩子的生活,而且为孩子价值观的建设也打下了良好的基础。

三、心理护理

1.杜绝指责 即使孩子犯了错,也有比指责更好的教育方法。尽量不要用否定的词句去教育孩子,会打击他们活动的主动性。

2.建立规矩 1~3 岁幼儿总会冒出一些"大不敬"的话,抚养者不要因为好玩而一笑了之,要严重地告知他们,这样说是不对的,没有规矩不成方圆,尽快纠正他们。否则以后你的生活中就会多个没礼貌、讨人嫌的"小麻烦"。

3.约束行为　1~3岁幼儿有时会向大人提出一些不合理的要求。抚养者要对他们的要求慎重地对待,让幼儿明白,每个人都应该约束自己的行为,不是什么都可以做的。

4.父母教养意见一致　教养幼儿的时候,大人要保持一致意见,切不可出现红脸和白脸角色分化,尽量不要有意见分歧。

5.培养幼儿的爱心　对于1~3岁幼儿的主要抚养者,必须本身具有一颗仁慈的心,给他们建立榜样的示范作用,这样方便幼儿能模仿和体验到父母的爱心,并能逐渐获得爱心。

6.培养信念　幼儿虽然还谈不上信念,但是必须让他自己有幼稚的计划和想要实现的愿望,愿意为此花费时间和精力,父母也要对他们的愿望进行相应满足,要予以鼓励。

练习题

1.幼儿期年龄阶段为(　　　　)
　　A.0~1岁　　　　　　　　B.1~3岁　　　　　　　C.4~8岁　　　　　　　D.10~15岁

2.埃里克森认为幼儿期的主要发展任务是(　　　　)
　　A.获得勤奋感,克服自卑感　　　　　　　　B.获得主动感,克服内疚感
　　C.获得自主感,克服羞耻感　　　　　　　　D.获得亲密感,避免孤独感

3.儿童哪个时期接受如厕训练效果最佳(　　　　)
　　A.婴儿时期　　　　　　　B.幼儿时期　　　　　　C.小学时期　　　　　　D.中学时期

4.幼儿期儿童的主导活动是(　　　　)
　　A.饮食　　　　　　　　　B.睡眠　　　　　　　　C.游戏　　　　　　　　D.学习

5.下列哪个时期是儿童口头言语发展的关键期(　　　　)
　　A.婴儿末期　　　　　　　B.幼儿期　　　　　　　C.小学低年级　　　　　D.小学中年级

6.幼儿体验高自尊与以后生活中哪项表项有关(　　　　)
　　A.不能很好地适应学校生活　　　　　　　　B.压抑或焦虑等不良情绪
　　C.对生活的满意度和幸福感下降　　　　　　D.缺乏人际交往能力

参考答案

第五章　学龄前期儿童的发展

第一节　学龄前期儿童的生理发展

一、身体发展

这个阶段,身高和体重呈波浪式上升,2 岁以后,生长速度逐渐缓慢,平均每年身高增长 4 ~ 5 cm,体重增加 5 ~ 6 kg。骨骼发育快,大约有 45 个新骨骺,即软骨变为骨骺的生长点。生殖系统 4 岁开始发育减缓,直至青少年期快速发育。循环系统中淋巴组织生长速度非常快,到青少年期下降(淋巴组织有助于抗感染、促进营养吸收,利于儿童健康和生存)。消化系统方面,2 岁半出齐 20 颗乳牙,到幼儿晚期,乳牙开始脱落;胃容量小,营养摄取应丰富且高质量。

二、大脑发育

此时脑重达到成人的 90%,前额叶快速发育,小脑功能逐渐加强,高级神经活动中,自主神经发育不完全。前额叶快速发展。小脑功能逐渐加强,能准确地协调进行各种动作,很好地维持身体平衡。3 岁,肌肉活动的协调性明显增强;5 ~ 6 岁,能准确协调地进行各种动作。高级神经活动——兴奋占优势,抑制过程不够完善,兴奋过程强于抑制过程。好动,容易激动,注意力不集中,容易受外界刺激而转移;兴奋过程加强,睡眠时间逐渐减少;抑制过程加强,学会控制自己的行为和较精确地进行各种活动。自主神经发育不完全,交感神经兴奋性强而副交感神经兴奋性较弱,心率及呼吸频率较快,但节律不稳定。幼儿肠胃消化能力极易受情绪影响。

三、运动发展

学龄前期儿童身体发展迅速,运动能力大幅度提高。此阶段儿童能够平衡身体,双脚连续向前跳;能够进行单杠悬垂动作 10 s 左右;能够较为轻松地完成 15 m 跑;能用单手投掷,将沙包向前投

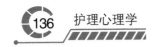

掷 2 m 左右;双脚跳、单脚跳时会弯曲上身;能够双手向上抛球;能够完成 1 km 左右的独立行走(途中可适当休息);能够以单脚连续向前跳 2 m 左右,左、右脚皆能单脚跳,可以双脚交替上下楼梯;会自己吃饭、刷牙、洗脸;学会自己穿套头衣服、扣扣子、拉拉链;能练习拍球,能伸手接球,会对准目标丢球、踢球。

第二节　学龄前期儿童的认知发展

一、语言发展

儿童心理的研究成果和长期的教育实践已经证明,幼儿期是人掌握语言最迅速的时期,也是最关键的时期。3~4 岁孩子的语言发展很大程度上取决于外界的环境刺激,取决于教育的影响。为儿童创设家庭式温馨、宽松的语言环境是发展儿童语言的一个重要前提。

3~4 岁是孩子语言发展最关键的时期,提高孩子的语言表达能力是一项艰巨任务。在教育工作中,要为孩子创设丰富多彩的生活环境,给孩子一个自由的家庭式语言氛围。利用文学作品培养孩子良好的早期阅读习惯更是一种重要的教育方式。孩子在温馨、自由的语言环境中,其语言的各方面能力及兴趣才能得到更好的发展。

二、注意力发展特点

4 岁孩子的注意力是能通过培养而加强的,在学龄前教育中应注意以下几点。

1. 明确学习目的　孩子对学习的目的性越明确,注意力越容易持久。

2. 培养兴趣　当孩子对某项内容发生兴趣时,注意力容易集中而且持久,故学龄前教育的形式应多样化、形象生动。

3. 创建良好的学习环境　学习时要尽量保持室内外安静,成人不要在屋内多走动,不要和孩子讲与学习内容无关的话。

三、想象力发展特点

4 岁的孩子,其想象力总的来说是贫乏的、简单的,缺乏明确的目的,以无意想象为主,有意想象和创造想象正在逐步发展,但不占主导地位。无意想象主要特点如下。

1. 想象主题多变　想象的主题多变,不能按一定目的进行下去,容易从一个主题转到另一个主题。例如一会儿想当一名医生,一会儿又想当警察。

2. 想象与现实无法区分　想象与现实分不开,不能把想象的事物跟现实的事物清楚地区分开来,因此,常被人家误认为说谎。例如他喜欢汽车玩具,就把其他小孩子的汽车想象成自己的,说这辆汽车是我的。

3. 想象具有特殊的夸大性　喜欢夸大事物的某些特征或情节。例如问小孩子你希望长得多高,他会回答"长得像天空一样高"。

四、思维的发展

皮亚杰认为 2~7 岁儿童思维属于前运算阶段,这是儿童克服各种心理障碍逐渐向逻辑思维过渡的时期。这一阶段儿童主要是表象性思维,思维的基本特点就是相对具体性、不可逆性、自我中心性和刻板性。

第三节　学龄前期儿童的心理发展

一、主动对内疚的冲突

在这一时期如果儿童表现出的主动探究行为受到鼓励,儿童就会形成主动性,这为他将来成为一个有责任感、有创造力的人奠定了基础。如果成人讥笑儿童的独创行为和想象力,那么儿童就会逐渐失去自信心,这使他们更倾向于生活在别人为他们安排好的狭窄圈子里,缺乏自己开创幸福生活的主动性。

当儿童的主动感超过内疚感时,他们就有了"目的"的品质。埃里克森把目的定义为:"一种正视和追求有价值目标的勇气,这种勇气不为儿童想象的失利、罪疚感和惩罚的恐惧所限制。"

二、自我意识的发展

在教育的影响下,儿童自我意识有了进一步的发展。相关研究表明,儿童自我意识各因素发展总趋势随年龄的增长而增长。

1. 自我概念的发展　7 岁以前,儿童对自己的描绘仅限于身体特征、年龄、性别和喜爱的活动等,还不会描述内部心理特征。儿童早期的认知能力处于具体形象思维阶段,他们很容易把自我、身体与心理混淆起来。儿童的概念是"物理概念",儿童对内在的心理体验和外在的物理体验不加区分。

2. 自我评价的发展　自我评价的能力在 3 岁儿童中还不明显,自我评价开始发生转折的年龄是3.5 ~ 4.0 岁,此年龄段的发展速度较 4 ~ 5 岁时要快,5 岁儿童绝大多数已能进行自我评价。

此期儿童自我评价的特点如下。

(1)从轻信成人的评价到自己独立评价。

(2)从对外部行为的评价到对内心品质的评价。

(3)从比较笼统的评价到比较细致的评价。

总的来说,学龄前期儿童的自我评价能力还很差,成人对学龄前期儿童的评价在儿童个性发展中起影响作用。因此,成人必须善于对儿童做出适当的评价,对儿童行为做过高或过低的评价对儿童都是有害的。

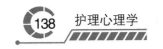

第四节　学龄前期儿童的情绪发展

一、移情能力迅速发展

4~5岁的儿童已具有较强的移情能力,能将自己置身于他人处境,设身处地为他人着想,接受他人的情感。有移情能力的儿童,更倾向于将移情唤起转变为对悲伤者的关心,最终促进利他行为的发展。如,当孩子看到一个同伴因损坏而失去了一个有趣的玩具而感到悲伤时,他会想到,如果自己失去了这样的玩具,也会悲伤。这时的悲伤是自我中心的移情,将同伴的情境移到自己身上。同时他也会想到,他是我的同伴,他悲伤,所以我也悲伤,并应该帮助和安慰他。此外,由于语言的发展,4~5岁儿童学会了更多的表达情绪的词语,例如高兴、害怕、难受、生气、喜欢、恨、爱、讨厌等,他们经常利用这些情绪词语描述自己和别人的情绪体验,他们也能用各种情绪性语言去安抚别人或影响别人的行为。

二、情绪理解依存于社会知识

4~5岁是儿童情绪理解能力发展的关键期。这个时期的儿童对情绪的理解处于社会知识依存型阶段,他们更倾向于根据已有的社会知识对他人的情绪做出刻板的推测并做出相应的行为反应。4~5岁儿童能够运用社会行为规范并初步评价自己的行为,还能在成人的帮助下,调控自己的行为,自制能力开始形成,有初步的责任感、道德感。儿童人际关系也发生重大变化,向同龄人关系过渡,能关心他人的情感反应,关心同伴,能友好合作,体验自己内在心理活动。但是这个时期的儿童在认知和情感上都还较以自我为中心,容易以自己的想法去推断他人的情绪情感,在认识他人情绪、管理他人情绪方面的能力较弱。

第五节　学龄前期儿童健康评估和护理

学龄前期儿童的活动范围扩大,智力发展快,自理能力增强,机体抵抗力逐渐增强,但仍易患小儿传染病。保健重点:继续进行生长发育监测;加强早期教育,培养独立生活能力和良好的道德品质;加强体格锻炼,增强体质;防治传染病,防止意外发生;加强托幼机构的管理。

保健的具体措施如下。

一、营养

学龄前期儿童饮食接近成人,每日三餐,可有2~3次加餐。儿童食欲受活动和情绪的影响较大。增进食欲的方法包括进食前让其休息几分钟,进餐时保持愉快、宽松的气氛,使用其喜欢的餐具和舒适的桌椅等。成人应为儿童树立健康饮食习惯和良好进餐礼仪的榜样。学龄前期儿童喜欢参与食物的制作和餐桌的布置,家长可利用此机会进行营养知识、食品卫生和防止烫伤等健康教育。

二、日常活动

学龄前期儿童已有自我照顾的能力,他们在学习自己进食、洗脸、刷牙等自理行为时,虽然动作缓慢、不协调,常需他人帮助,这样可能会花费成人更多的时间和精力,但应给予其鼓励,使他们能更独立。学龄前期儿童每日睡 11 ~ 12 h。此期儿童想象力极其丰富,因此夜间常有怕黑和做噩梦的现象。家长需安抚孩子,可在室内开一盏小灯。入睡前可与孩子做一些轻松、愉快的活动以减轻紧张情绪。学龄前期儿童十分活跃,他们从日常游戏和活动中可以得到较多锻炼。保健人员还应指导家长在孩子体格锻炼时充分利用空气、日光和水,开展三浴锻炼。

三、保护牙齿

重视乳牙龋病。牙齿清洁不干净会导致乳牙龋病,若治疗不及时,会严重影响恒牙生长。若恒牙萌出而出现双层牙时,应把乳牙拔掉,否则会令牙齿排列不整、咬合不正。饮食过于精细,会导致牙齿咀嚼功能下降,颌骨发育较差。应当保证孩子营养均衡,并让孩子改掉舔牙齿等坏习惯。舔牙等坏习惯会造成牙列不齐等畸形现象,影响牙齿功能和面部美观。要特别注意的是牙齿的保养,保持口腔清洁,坚持早、晚刷牙,饭后漱口。

练习题

1. 以下属于学龄前期儿童的年龄阶段是(　　)
　 A. 0 ~ 1 岁
　 B. 1 ~ 3 岁
　 C. 4 ~ 6 岁
　 D. 7 ~ 10 岁

2. 4 ~ 5 岁属于弗洛伊德理论中的(　　)
　 A. 口唇期
　 B. 肛门期
　 C. 性器期
　 D. 潜伏期

3. 4 ~ 5 岁孩子帮忙做家务就鼓励他,属于埃里克森人格发展理论中哪项冲突(　　)
　 A. 获得勤奋感,克服自卑感
　 B. 获得主动感,克服内疚感
　 C. 获得自主感,克服羞耻感
　 D. 获得信任感,克服不信任感

4. 下列不是受欢迎儿童的特点是(　　)
　 A. 学习成绩好
　 B. 安静,有顺从性
　 C. 善于交往,易于合作
　 D. 独立活动能力强,有主见

5. 埃里克森认为学龄前期良好的人格特征是(　　)
　 A. 希望品质
　 B. 意志品质
　 C. 目标品质
　 D. 能力品质

参考答案

第六章　学龄期儿童的发展

━━━━━━ 学习目标 ━━━━━━

1. 掌握学龄期儿童护理工作。
2. 熟悉学龄期儿童心理、认知、社会和情感发展的特点。
3. 了解学龄期儿童生理发展的特点。

7~13 岁是儿童开始进入小学学习的时期。这是儿童心理发展的一个重要转折时期。在小学低年级,儿童还具有明显的学龄前儿童的心理特点,而小学高年级儿童则随着生理年龄的变化,逐渐步入青春发育期。因此,小学时期往往被称为前青春发育期。

学龄期儿童的心理处于快速、协调发展的时期,学龄期是促进智力发展、形成和谐个性、培养良好心理品质与行为习惯的好时机。

第一节　学龄期儿童的生理发展

学龄期儿童的大脑结构得到迅速发展,12 岁儿童为 1 400 g,达到成人的水平。7 岁儿童平均睡眠时间 11 h,10 岁平均为 10 h,12 岁儿童平均为 9~10 h。12 岁以后,孩子的智能发展基本就定型了。低年级学生一般为 6~8 岁,在生理上处于平稳发展的时期。骨骼肌肉茁壮成长,特别是下肢骨骼的增长,比身体增长还要快。但肌肉发育尚不完全,含水分多,肌肉纤维较细,肌腱宽而短,关节的软骨较厚,关节囊韧带薄而松弛,关节周围肌肉较细长,关节的伸展性活动范围较大,牢固性较差,容易发生脱臼。同时血液循环比较快,心率较快,应防止心脏负担过重和体力活动过度。大肌肉动作的协调性比幼儿期有很大的发展,但小肌肉动作的协调性还较差。比如,一年级的学生写字时,不仅速度慢而且不工整。这一阶段的儿童,不宜做强度太大、时间太久的体育运动,在训练写字、弹琴等这些小肌肉运动的动作时,要注意动作的规范性。

三四年级学生一般为 8~10 岁,总的说来,身体发育处于相对平稳阶段。除大脑外,三四年级学生的各项生理指标只在量上比一二年级学生有所提高,基本没有质的飞跃,仍处于平稳发展的时期。男女生体质性的差别明显,女生发育早于男生。三四年级学生肌肉中含水率较高,肌肉细长而且柔嫩。三四年级学生的心脏容积和血管容积之比小于高年级。三四年级学生神经系统发展较快,兴奋和抑制的功能有所增强,每日平均需睡眠的时间为 10 h 左右,清醒时间增多,控制和调节自己行为的能力提高较明显。

五六年级学生一般为 10~12 岁,总的说来,身体发育处于增长率高峰阶段。五六年级学生身体素质指标均有提高,短跑成绩男生优于女生,灵敏素质发展也极为快速,学习和掌握技术动作较快。

五六年级学生的心脏仍具有学龄前儿童的特点,脉搏频率较快,但心脏发育十分显著,已接近青春期的特点。因此,适当加大运动量,会使学生的心脏容积和心脏功能得到显著发展。11~12岁儿童脑的重量已接近成年人的水平,大脑活动的功能有显著提高,兴奋功能也增强了,11~12岁平均睡眠9 h即可。五六年级学生,身体发育再次进入一个高速发展期,被称为第二发展期。此时,他们不仅身高、体重明显增长,而且肌肉骨骼的力量也在迅速增强,特别是到六年级的时候,第二性征开始出现。

第二节　学龄期儿童的心理发展

一、勤奋与自卑的冲突

这一阶段的儿童都应在学校接受教育。学校是训练儿童适应社会、掌握今后生活所必需的知识和技能的地方。如果他们能顺利地完成学习课程,他们就会获得勤奋感,这使他们在今后的独立生活和承担工作任务中充满信心;反之,就会产生自卑感。另外,如果儿童养成了过分看重自己的工作的态度,而对其他方面木然处之,这种人的生活是可悲的。埃里克森说:"如果他把工作当成他唯一的任务,把做什么工作看成是唯一的价值标准,那他就可能成为自己工作技能和老板们最驯服和最无思想的奴隶。"

当儿童的勤奋感大于自卑感时,他们就会获得有"能力"的品质。埃里克森说:"能力是不受儿童自卑感削弱的,完成任务所需要的是自由操作的熟练技能和智慧。"

二、学龄期儿童的认知发展

(一)学龄期儿童思维能力的发展

1.概括能力发展　这种发展表现在儿童能从对事物外部特点的概括(形象概括)发展到对事物本质属性的概括(抽象概括);从对简单事物的概括发展到对复杂事物的概括。学龄期儿童的概括能力是随年龄的增长而逐渐发展的,但发展的过程有时快有时慢,对不同事物的认知发展是不同步的。

2.比较能力发展　从事物相异点到相同点的比较,从具体事物的异同到抽象事物的异同,从直观比较到用词语在头脑中比较。研究表明,学龄期儿童比较能力的发展表现在:从区分具体事物的异同,逐渐发展到区分许多部分关系的异同;从直接感知条件下的比较逐步发展到运用语言在头脑中引起表象的条件下进行比较。学龄期儿童的比较不是在所有条件下都是相同的,对某些事物的比较既能找出相似点又能找出细微的差别,但在另一些条件下,他们进行比较时则有不同。

(二)学龄期儿童的学习特点

1.学习是学龄期儿童的主导活动　学校学习是在教师指导下,有目的、系统地掌握知识、技能和行为规范的活动。儿童在这种特殊的学习过程中习得知识、技能,掌握社会责任感和义务感。

2.教和学是师生双向互动的过程　教师的教是传授知识过程中答疑、解惑、育人,学生是积极主动的学习者,而不应被视为是被动的接受者。教和学是师生双方积极主动的互动过程。

(三)学龄期儿童社会发展特点

社会性是在个体社会化过程中发展起来的,与社会存在相适应的一切特征和典型的行为方式的总和。

1. **亲子交往** 儿童入学以后,与父母的关系发生了很大变化。表现为儿童与父母的交往时间、交往内容和交往方式都有所改变。在交往时间上,与学龄前期相比学龄期儿童与父母在一起的时间相对减少,父母关注儿童的时间也相对减少,儿童对父母的依恋和依赖程度减弱。在交往内容上,学龄期儿童的父母更多关注孩子学业和品德,如辅导学习、检查作业、与孩子讨论学校里发生的事情、讨论日常行为举止的适当性等。在交往方式上,父母的控制性在小学阶段开始减弱。研究表明,随着儿童年龄的增长,儿童越来越多地自己做决定,6 岁以前儿童的大部分事情是由父母决定的。

2. **同伴交往与同伴团体的形成** 同伴交往是儿童形成和发展个性特点,形成社会行为、价值观和态度的一个独特的社会化方式。同伴交往的特点主要表现为:与同伴交往的时间更多,交往的形式更为复杂;在同伴交往中传递信息的技能增强,他们能够更好地理解他人的动机和目的,能更好地对他人进行反馈,其同伴间的交流更加有效;他们更善于利用各种信息来决定自己对他人采取的行动;更善于协调与其他儿童的交往活动;开始形成同伴团体。

第三节 学龄期儿童情绪和性格发展

一、学龄期儿童的情绪发展

随着年龄的逐渐增长以及生命体验的丰富,学龄期儿童情感的内容不断丰富,情感进一步分化,表现情感的方法也越来越丰富。他们情感的深刻性不断增加,对于事情的归因能力不断增强,更加趋于现实化。情绪的稳定性和可控性明显增强,他们不再像学前阶段那样易冲动,逐渐能够控制自己的情绪。而且在这一阶段儿童的道德感和理智感逐渐发展,逐渐能够对行为做出一定的判断,好奇心也越来越强,对学习和生活产生广泛的兴趣。

二、学龄期儿童的性格发展

所谓性格,是指个体对现实的稳定态度以及与之相适应的行为方式中所表现出来的个性心理特征,主要表现在个体对现实的态度和个体的行为方式中。学龄期儿童正处在性格的形成期,这个时期的儿童虽然初步具有独立处理事情的能力,但还极易接受社会环境的熏染,尤其是家庭的影响。因为处在性格的形成期,学龄期儿童性格的态度特征不稳定,经常左右摇摆。学龄期儿童的理智特征在二年级到四年级时稳定发展,而四年级到六年级时会出现一个迅速发展时期。学龄期儿童的情绪特征不断发展,其中情绪的强度和持久性发展较快,因为六年级儿童刚刚进入青春期,其行为特别容易受到情绪的影响。从性格的意志特征来讲,学龄期儿童的自制力和坚持性都呈现下降趋势。原因是低年级儿童受外部控制,随年龄增长,对外部控制的依赖减少,但内部控制又还没有发展起来,不足以调节和控制自己。

第四节 学龄期儿童身心护理

针对学龄期儿童护理工作,主要从身体和心理两大方面进行。

一、身体护理

学龄期是儿童成长发育的黄金时期,所需要的营养元素也会更多,需要吃更多营养丰富的食物帮助其成长。对于学龄期儿童来说,需要多吃一些蛋白质、维生素以及钙含量丰富的食物,才能满足身体的营养需求,更好地成长。因为进入学习阶段,需要养成规律生活作息,因此要重视儿童的早餐和课间加餐。补充牛奶、核桃仁、鱼类等物质,牛奶不仅含有丰富的蛋白质,还含有很多钙、磷等矿物质,不仅有利于生长发育,而且对身高最为关键的骨骼生长有好处。核桃仁有很多的营养,它不仅包含大量的脂肪酸,能降低身体炎症反应,预防心血管疾病,还有助于控制糖尿病。核桃仁中含有的锰有助于强化骨骼,镁有助于器官、肌肉、神经系统的正常工作。鱼类富含身体所必需的维生素 B_1,还有很多的蛋白质可以增强人体的抵抗力,多吃鱼类还有助于大脑的健康,能提高人体的记忆力。

二、心理护理

小学阶段不仅是基础教育的初始阶段,还是学生初步体验知识、获得知识和掌握技能的关键时期。在小学期间,学生要拥有正确的学习态度、良好的学习习惯等,才能为未来的学习生活打下牢固的基础。但是在步入小学初期时,由于跳跃式的改变,部分小学低年级学生出现学习适应不良的现象,从而导致学生学习成绩下降、缺乏学习兴趣等问题。家长应激发学习兴趣,提高学习效率。孔子说过:"知之者不如好之者,好之者不如乐之者。"学习兴趣是保持良好注意力能力的核心要素,也是学习的强大动力。一旦激发学生的学习兴趣,学生的学习效率将会不断提高。小学低年级学生具有好动、充满好奇、爱模仿和可塑性强的年龄特点,会对新奇的事物感兴趣,应遵循学生年龄特点,因材施教。著名教育家朱熹曾说过:"圣贤施教,各因其材,小以小成,大以大成,无弃人也。"实施因材施教,要求教师要从实际出发,尊重学生现有的身心发展情况,学会从不同的角度促进小学低年级学生德、智、体、美、劳各方面发展。在教学过程中,教师不但要将教育落实到全体学生的身上,同时也不放弃后进生,要时刻抓住每一个学生身上的闪光点。

练习题

1. 学龄期儿童年龄阶段是(　　　)
　A. 0～1 岁　　　　　　B. 1～3 岁　　　　　　C. 4～5 岁　　　　　　D. 7～12 岁
2. 学龄期亲子关系的变化表现为(　　　)
　A. 直接交往的时间明显增加　　　　　B. 父母教养关注重点的转移
　C. 儿童尚无自主管理的能力　　　　　D. 父母对儿童的控制力量逐渐加强
3. 对待学龄期儿童,最应该注意他的(　　　)
　A. 感情问题　　　　B. 入学适应问题　　　　C. 亲情问题　　　　D. 压力问题
4. 根据埃里克森人格发展理论,学龄期儿童具体冲突为(　　　)
　A. 信任对不信任　　　B. 主动对内疚　　　C. 勤奋对自卑　　　D. 亲密对孤独

参考答案

第七章　青少年的发展

▨▨▨▨▨ 学习目标 ▨▨▨▨▨

1. 掌握青少年自我意识、情绪、道德和人际交往等方面的表现及发展特点;青少年身心护理工作。
2. 熟悉青少年个性和社会性发展的一般特点。
3. 了解青少年身心发展的一般特点。

第一节　青少年的生理发展

青春期是童年向成年过渡的时期,在这一时期,青少年在生理和心理上都产生了巨大的变化,是个体身体发展的鼎盛时期及性成熟时期。生理上的成熟使青少年在心理上产生成人感,他们希望能获得成人的某些权利,找到新的行为标准并渴望变换社会角色。然而,由于他们的心理发展水平有限,有许多期望不能实现,容易产生挫折感。总之,由于此阶段身心发展不平衡,使青少年面临种种心理危机,并出现一些心理及行为问题。

青少年身体发展主要表现为身高、体重的急剧增长以及第二性征的发育。进入青年初期后,个体逐渐达到性成熟,青少年的心、肺、脑和神经系统等也继续发育,这些生理发育过程在青年初期结束时基本完成。

青春期是个体生长发育的第二个高峰期,主要表现在身体外形的变化、体内生理功能的增强以及性的发育和成熟3个方面,这就是青春期生理发育的三大巨变。

一、身体外形的变化

青春期的少年身体发育很快,其身高、体重及面部特征等都发生了很大变化,这些变化使他们在外形上逐渐接近成人。

1. 身高的增长　青春期的少年外形变化最明显的特征就是身高的迅速增长。人身高的增长有两个高峰,第一个高峰发生在1岁左右,那时身高一般增加50%以上;第二次生长高峰就出现于青春期,在这个阶段,青少年身高增长异常迅速。

2. 体重的增长　青少年在体重方面也有较大的发展变化。从我国城乡男女青少年体重增长曲线可以看出,男孩在12~14岁这段时间,体重增加最快,平均每年增长5.0 kg,13岁是增长高峰,15岁以后增长速度迅速下降。女孩在11~13岁时体重增加最快,平均每年增长4.5 kg,11~12岁是增长高峰,13岁后增长速度迅速下降。

3.第二性征的出现　第二性征是性发育的外部表现,是青少年身体外形变化的重要标志。随着第二性征的出现,青少年开始从童年的中性状态进入到两性分化的状态。在男性身上,第二性征主要表现为喉结突出、嗓音低沉、体格高大、肌肉发达、唇部出现胡须、周身出现多而密的汗毛、出现腋毛和阴毛等。在女性身上,第二性征则表现为嗓音细润、乳房隆起、骨盆宽大、皮下脂肪较多、臀部变大、体态丰满、出现腋毛和阴毛等。这些第二性征的出现使得男女青少年在外形上的差异日益明显。

二、体内生理功能的增强

在青春发育期,个体体内的各种生理功能都在迅速增强并逐渐达到成熟。

1.心脏压缩功能的增强　青春期少年的心血管系统出现了一些新的功能特点。形态上,为了保证青春期生长发育的需要,作为人体运输系统的心血管系统也出现了第二次生长加速。在9岁时,儿童的心脏重量为出生时的6倍,在青春期开始后,则增长至12～14倍;同样,心脏密度也在青春期成倍地增长。而且,由于青春期少年活动量的增加,构成心室壁的肌肉增厚,心肌纤维更富有弹力,这就为心脏每次收缩时能压挤出更多血液创造了条件。在机制方面,主要表现为心率、脉率开始减慢。这一方面是因为支配心脏活动的神经纤维已发育健全,能更有效地调节心脏活动,另一方面则是由于心脏本身功能的增强,使每次心搏所排出的血量增多,每分钟只需搏动70～80次便能满足机体的需求。

2.肺的发育　在青春期,肺的发育也明显加速。12岁左右,肺重量为出生时的10倍,肺小叶结构逐渐完善,肺泡容量增大,与呼吸有关的某些肌肉发育加快,使呼吸功能进一步加强。在整个青春期,肺活量将比青春期前增加1倍多。男女肺活量存在显著的差异。

3.肌肉力量的增强　青春期少年体重的增加表明肌肉和骨骼发生了变化。在肌肉力量的发展水平上,男女之间也存在着明显的差异。

4.大脑的发育　在量的方面,青春期少年脑重及脑容量的增长不显著,因为儿童在10岁以前,其脑重已为成人的95%。但在质的方面,这时脑的发展则有较大进展。我国脑电波的相关研究表明,个体在4～20岁存在2个脑发展的加速期,第一个发生在5～6岁,第二个发生在13岁左右,即青春期。神经系统也基本上与成人没有什么差异了,大脑皮质沟回组合完善,神经纤维完成髓鞘化。随着脑和神经系统的发育成熟,青少年大脑的兴奋和抑制也逐渐趋于平衡。

三、性的发育和成熟

生殖系统是人体各系统中发育成熟最晚的,它的成熟标志着人体生理发育的完成。

1.性激素的增多　性激素分泌是整个内分泌系统活动的一个重要内容。在青春期以前,无论男女,都仅分泌少量的性激素。进入青春期后,个体下丘脑的促性腺激素释放激素的分泌量增加,从而使垂体前叶的促性腺激素分泌也增加,进而导致性腺激素水平相应提高,促进性腺发育。女性的性腺为卵巢,男性的性腺为睾丸。性腺的发育成熟使女性出现月经,男性发生遗精。

2.性器官的发育　女性的性器官包括卵巢、子宫及阴道。在青春期前发育缓慢,8～10岁发育加快,以后的发育速度则呈直线上升。子宫的发育从10岁始到18岁止。长度增加了1倍,其形状及各部分的比例也有所改变。

男性的性器官包括睾丸、附睾、精囊、前列腺及阴茎。男性的性器官发育比女性要晚些,在10岁以前发育很慢,进入青春期后发育加速。

第二节　青少年的心理发展

随着青少年生理和智力所发生的一系列特殊的变化,他们在心理发展上也出现了许多新特点,表现在自我意识、情绪情感、日常心态以及与父母同伴的关系等诸多方面。总体来讲,青少年的个性特点有二:其一是不平衡性;其二是极端性或偏执性。

一、自我意识的发展

(一)自我意识的基本特点

青春期是自我意识发展的第二个飞跃期。在个体进入青春期以前,曾出现过一次自我意识发展的飞跃期,年龄在 1~3 岁,以儿童可以用代词"我"来标志自己为重要特点。在接下来的若干年里,儿童的自我意识虽然还在继续发展着,但发展的速度则是相对平稳的。

进入青春期后,由于身体的迅速发育,青少年很快出现了成人的体貌特征。因为这种生理上的变化发生得过于突然,使他们在产生一种惶惑感觉的同时,自觉或不自觉地将自己的思想从一直嬉戏于其中的客观世界中抽回了很大一部分,重新指向主观世界,使思想意识再一次进入自我,从而导致自我意识的第二次飞跃。自我意识高涨的突出表现是,青少年的内心世界越发丰富起来,他们在日常生活和学习中,常常将很多心智用于内省。"我到底是个怎么样的人?""我的特征是什么?""别人喜欢我还是讨厌我?"等一系列关于"我"的问题开始反复萦绕于他们的心中,这种倾向在其作文及日记中常可以清楚地观察到。例如,同是以"我看到了什么"为内容的作文,小学生是纯粹地描述客观世界的景象,而青少年虽然仍对客观世界进行描述,但在他们的描述中却带有浓重的个人情绪情感基调,在作文中更突出了个人的喜好、烦恼和憧憬等。

青春期自我意识高涨的另一个主要表现是其个性上的主观偏执性。一方面,他们总是认为自己正确,听不进别人的意见;另一方面,他们又感到别人似乎总是用挑剔的态度对待他们。因此,当听到别人在低声讲话,便断定是在议论自己;当看到别人面露微笑,又认为是在嘲笑自己;如果某位老师多看了自己一眼,就会认为是自己做错了什么……

(二)自我概念

个性的形成也包括具有相对稳定的自我概念或自我形象。一个人是否具有一个适当的自我概念对其个性的发展至关重要。

青少年期个体的认知能力有了很大的提高,他们能以更加抽象、复杂和独特的方式来认识自己,因此青少年的自我概念在内容和结构上都与早期个体的自我概念有很大的差异。这种差异主要表现在以下几个方面。

1. 自我概念更加抽象　皮亚杰的理论认为,个体在 11 或 12 岁的时候从具体运算思维向形式运算思维转变。进入青春期的个体已经不再用很具体的词语(如"我喜欢食物")描述他们的特征,而是更经常用概括性的词语来描述(如"我是一个真正的人")。到了青年早期,个体的自我概念则更抽象,不仅关注人格特点,同时也关注重要的价值观和意识形态及信念(如"我是一个伪自由主义者")。

2. 自我概念更加具有整合性和组织性　青少年期的个体在进行自我描述时,不仅仅像早期儿童一样列出自我各方面的特点,而且将自我知觉包括那些看起来是互相矛盾的方面整合成更具有逻辑性和连贯性的统一体。

3.自我概念的结构更加分化　青少年不再像儿童期个体那样概括地使用某些特质描述自己，而是认识到了自我在不同的情境下会有不同的表现。例如，青少年会区分自己父母、同伴以及恋人等不同交往对象来对自我进行描述，而且他们也会根据自己的不同社会角色分化出不同的自我概念。

（三）自我评价

自我评价指个体对自身的思想、能力、水平等方面所作的评价，它是自我调节机制的主要成分。自我评价的能力只有在青年早期才开始成熟。虽然个体在童年时就开始产生了一些简单的自我评价，但那时的自我评价多是由别人的态度和反应折射到自身而产生的，缺少内省性。到了青年早期，由于抽象逻辑思维的进一步发展、知识经验的日益丰富，青少年逐渐学会了较为全面、客观、辩证地看待自己、分析自己，自我评价的能力才变得全面、主动，而且日趋深刻。主要表现在他们不仅能分析自己一时的思想矛盾和心理状态，能认识到自己对某一具体行为起支配作用的个别心理特点，还能经常对自己的整个心理面貌进行估量，能认识到自己较为稳定的个性心理品质。

二、情绪发展特点

青少年的情绪表现充分体现出半成熟、半幼稚的矛盾性特点。随着青少年心理能力的发展和生活经验的扩大，其情绪的感受和表现形式不再像以往那么单一了，但还远不如成人的情绪体验那么稳定，表现出明确的两面性。

三、人际交往特点

在和同伴的关系上，青少年和儿童有明显的不同，主要表现在以下几个方面。

1.逐渐克服了团体的交往方式　儿童在结交朋友方面最明显的特点是结伴现象，表现为六七个儿童经常在一起交往和游戏。在这种交往中，他们感到了身心自由和愉快。因此，就交友的方式来说，小学时代是结伴的时代。到了小学高年级，这种交友的结伴形式发展到了顶点，然后趋于解体，被新的交往形式所取代。

2.朋友关系在青少年生活中日益重要　青少年对交朋友的意义也有了新的认识。他们认为朋友应该能够同甘苦、共患难，能够从对方那里得到支持和帮助。因此，他们对朋友的质量产生了特殊的要求，认为朋友应该坦率、通情达理、关心别人、保守秘密。在青少年的日常交往中，好朋友之间往往彼此公开自己认为最重要、最秘密的事情。这种交流对青少年的心理发展是有积极意义的，能够使他们通过别人更好地认识自己的内心世界，更好地了解自己。这一过程对其自我概念、观点采择和同一性的形成都有积极的作用。

观点和行动上的一致也是青少年朋友之间心理接近的重要条件之一。在某些场合下，好朋友之间经常要制订出一个一致的行动方针，若违反了方针就要受到严厉的谴责。他们认为，能否忠于协议、忠于朋友是衡量友谊的十分重要的尺度。

第三节　青少年的认知发展

根据皮亚杰的认知发展阶段理论可知，青少年正处于形式运算思维阶段（11岁及以上）。这个阶段的主要思维特点是，在头脑中可以把事物的形式和内容分开，可以离开具体事物，根据假设来进行逻辑推演，能运用形式运算来解决诸如组合、包含、比例、排除、概率及因素分析等逻辑课题。

青少年期的两个阶段:少年期和青年早期。少年期个体的形象思维趋于成熟,抽象逻辑思维开始占优势。从初中二年级开始,学生的抽象逻辑思维开始由经验型水平向理论型水平转化。因此初中生思维活动的基本特点是抽象逻辑思维已占优势地位,但有时思维中的具体形象成分还起作用。青年早期个体的形象思维已完全发展成熟,抽象逻辑思维的发展也进入了成熟期。到高中二年级时,经验型向理论型的转化初步完成,标志着他们的抽象逻辑思维趋向成熟。因此,逻辑思维的发展是青少年思维发展的重点。

按照思维中所遵循的逻辑规律与所用的逻辑方法的不同,逻辑思维可以分为形式逻辑思维和辩证逻辑思维两大类。形式逻辑思维和辩证逻辑思维也是抽象逻辑思维的两个不同的发展阶段,辩证逻辑思维是以形式逻辑思维为基础,且高于形式逻辑思维。这两种思维形式的发展和成熟,是青少年思维发展和成熟的重要标志。高中生形式逻辑思维的发展较为稳定而匀速,而辩证逻辑思维的发展则比较迅速。在此阶段,其形式逻辑思维获得了相当完善的发展,在思维活动中占据主导地位。而辩证逻辑思维的发展水平低于形式逻辑思维,两者的发展相辅相成,使得青少年的思维水平更高、更成熟、更完善。

随着年龄的增长,青少年的创造性思维水平总的趋势是不断向前发展的,年级越高,创造性思维水平越高,但发展速度是不均匀的,高二是创造性思维发展的高潮,初一和高三是创造性思维发展的低潮。随年龄的增长,高中生的创造性思维的流畅性呈下降趋势,变通性平稳发展,独特性逐渐提高。

除创造性想象和发散思维外,青少年创造性思维的发展还表现在顿悟、类比迁移及假设检验等方面。青少年个体的创造性思维处于高度发展阶段,个体创造性思维水平的高低对其创造力的表现有重要影响。

第四节　青少年的身心护理

一、心理护理

对于患病青少年,病床的安排,要尽量考虑青少年的年龄特点。尽量满足他们活泼好动的天性,为他们提供适当的空间并创造条件,使他们能够在住院期间心情愉快,安心接受治疗。当然,也有必要向他们讲清医院的有关规章制度以及疾病的有关知识、治疗方法等,使之积极配合治疗。

青少年处于发育阶段,生理上的第二性征的出现,往往使他们特别害羞。部分青少年不喜欢异性医务人员进行个别的健康指导和身体检查,但较易于接受年岁较大、较成熟的医生、护士的指导。渴望了解自己的病情,可是有时装作没兴趣,羞于启齿。这些都和青少年自身的心理特点有关,实际上是好强心理对渴望了解病情的心理的一种掩饰。因此,护士应洞察这一点,主动向他们做一些有关病情的解释和介绍,对治疗极有好处。

二、身体护理

1.培养良好生活习惯　合理安排生活、工作和学习,培养良好的卫生习惯,注意体格锻炼和适当的劳动。个人卫生包括口腔卫生、用眼卫生和写字、读书、站、坐等正确姿势,以防龋齿、近视眼和脊柱弯曲。按照不同年龄有计划地系统安排锻炼内容,顺序渐进。

2.保证睡眠　青春期睡眠时间 7~9 h,要养成良好的睡眠习惯。

3.**乳房保健** 少女到了青春期乳房隆起,应及时带上乳罩,但乳罩不要过紧或过松,过紧会影响乳房正常发育,过松则不能防止乳房下垂。

练习题

1. 人的记忆广度达到一生中的顶峰是在(　　)
   A. 幼儿期 　　　　　　　　　　B. 童年期
   C. 青春期 　　　　　　　　　　D. 青年期

2. 自我意识的第二次飞跃发生在(　　)
   A. 幼儿期 　　　　　　　　　　B. 青春期
   C. 青年期 　　　　　　　　　　D. 更年期

3. 第二逆反期主要发生在(　　)
   A.3~4 岁 　　　　　　　　　　B. 小学阶段
   C. 青春期 　　　　　　　　　　D. 青年期

4. 下列不属于帮助青少年顺利度过逆反期的重要内容是(　　)
   A. 父母要正确面对逆反期是个体心理发展过程必经的客观现象
   B. 父母必须正视青少年独立自主的需求
   C. 逆反期是青少年面临的心理社会问题
   D. 父母要认识青少年心理上的成人感与半成熟现状之间的矛盾是最基本的矛盾

5. 青春期的主要特点是(　　)
   A. 身心稳定 　　　　　　　　　B. 心理发展无显著变化
   C. 身心发展迅速而又不平衡 　　　D. 心理迅速发展并直达成熟

6. 下列关于青春期生理发育加速的描述,不正确的是(　　)
   A. 身体成长加速 　　　　　　　B. 生理功能发育加速
   C. 性的发育和成熟加速 　　　　D. 青春发育期提前

7. 按照埃里克森人格发展理论来讲,青春期遇到的冲突是(　　)
   A. 信任对不信任 　　　　　　　B. 主动对内疚
   C. 勤奋对自卑 　　　　　　　　D. 自我同一性对角色混乱

参考答案

第八章 成年早中期个体的发展

1. 掌握身体、心理和认知每个发展阶段的变化。
2. 熟悉成年早中期个体发展的基本问题。
3. 了解满足成年期个体健康活动的需求。

第一节 成年早期个体的概述

一、成年早期的年龄规定

个体从 11 岁到 19 岁,生理达到完全成熟。由此,从生理意义上,个体开始进入成年早期。在这里,我们将生理的成熟时间规定为成年早期的开始年龄(成年早期的上限),将社会生活的成熟时间规定为成年早期的结束,也就是成年中期的开始年龄(即成年早期的下限),据此将成年早期的年龄阶段规定为 19~40 岁。

二、成年早期的一般特征

成年早期在人的一生发展中具有重要意义,在这一时期,个体的身心发展趋于稳定成熟,智力发展达到全盛时期,建立起家庭并创立事业,开始全面适应社会生活。这一时期的个体有以下几方面的特征。

1. 从成长期到稳定期的变化 儿童及青少年阶段被称为成长期。青少年时期生理发展达到了高峰,心理也趋向初步成熟。进入成年早期后,个体进入稳定期。这种稳定性体现在绝大多数成年早期的个体身上,具体表现为:①生理发展趋于稳定;②心理发展,尤其是情感过程趋于成熟,性格特点基本定型;③生活方式趋于固定化和习惯化;④建立了较为稳定的家庭;⑤社会职业稳定,且能忠于职守。

2. 智力发展到达全盛时期 成年早期个体的智力发展进入全盛时期。思维方式由形式逻辑思维为主转为以辩证逻辑思维为主,思维更加具有相对性、灵活性、整合性和实用性。在成年早期的最后阶段,个体的创造性思维发展也达到高峰,开始在不同领域内表现出不同程度的创造力。

三、成年早期的认知特点

1. 成年早期智力发展 智力的发展是一个适应的过程。影响成年早期智力发展的重要因素之一,是个体所处的新的客观环境及所面临的新的适应任务。

在十八九岁以前,个体的主要任务是获取与社会文化有关的知识系统,以消除与社会之间的矛盾,达到对社会的适应,实现社会化。个体这时所处的客观环境是受成人保护的。进入成年早期以后,经过进一步的正规或非正规的学习,个体已基本掌握了本民族的文化系统及社会道德系统,对社会的基本要求已能适应,但此时又面临着社会生活的新的挑战,如事业、婚姻、家庭等,需要不断进行恰当的分析、判断、推理,达到对问题的解决。

2.成年早期智力一般特点　成年早期智力表现从总体水平来看,表现出相对稳定的特点。但与此同时,成年早期个体的智力在性质上仍表现出一些全新的属性。例如,个体在儿童和青少年期处于知识获取阶段。成年早期处于实现阶段,个体为了实现长远的目标,必须让自己的认知能力适应复杂的环境(如婚姻和工作)。在这个阶段个体减少了知识获取活动,而更多地关注在日常生活中应用所获取的知识。成年中期处于责任阶段,对应的是履行义务和责任。老年时期是知识的重新组合阶段。

3.成年早期记忆发展特点　在记忆力方面,对于成年早期的个体来说,虽然机械记忆能力有所下降,但成年早期的前一阶段是人生中逻辑记忆能力发展的高峰期,其有意记忆、理解记忆占据主导地位,而且记忆容量也很大。

4.成年早期想象发展特点　在想象力方面,成年早期个体想象中的合理成分及创造性成分明显增加,克服了前几个发展阶段中所表现出的想象的过于虚幻性,使想象更具实际功用。

第二节　成年中期个体的概述

成年中期,即中年期,一般指40~65岁这段时期。成年中期的年龄范围是相对的,不是一成不变的。这是因为随着生活和医疗条件的改善,人的平均寿命在不断延长,划分青年、中年、老年的年龄界限也随之变动;此外,在具体研究过程中,研究对象之间由于生活的自然条件、地理环境、生活方式、生活水平、个体修养等方面的不同,即使是年龄相同,其健康状态和衰老程度也有可能相差很大。

作为人生历程中的一个阶段,成年中期的个体无论是生理上还是心理上都发生了一系列变化。由于成年中期个体面临家庭、社会中的多种任务,担任着多种角色,个体的发展受到多种变量的共同影响,因此有关成年中期心理特点的研究难以得出统一的结论,成年中期也是目前研究较少的年龄阶段。

中年人是社会的中坚、家庭的核心,是物质财富和精神财富的主要创造者。因此,与人生历程其他阶段相比,中年人的家庭生活显得格外重要。

在个体人生历程的发展中,家庭是一个贯穿始终的重要的影响因素。个体受到这个小环境的影响,同时也对这个小环境产生影响。

家庭与个体生命一样,也有一个产生、发展与消亡的过程,并呈现出一定的周期性特点。所谓家庭生命周期,通常指的是从男女双方结为夫妻组成家庭开始,至夫妻双方死亡导致家庭解体而告终的家庭发展过程。根据家庭成员构成状况及发展任务的变化,家庭生命周期一般被划分为若干阶段。每一阶段都有相应的发展课题需要家庭成员去面对或解决。如何面对或解决这些发展课题,关系到家庭成员的心理发展进程与生活适应水平。

第三节　成年早中期个体护理和健康计划

一、心理护理

成年期由于家庭工作的繁重,负担、困难较多,情绪经常处于紧张状态,这个时期的心理卫生十分重要。

1. 协调各方面的人际关系　增强自我控制意识,在交往中应真诚、友好,避免非原则争议,对己严格、对人宽厚。良好的人际关系对生活和工作均有促进作用。

2. 家庭和睦、夫妻和谐　既是个人心身健康、生活幸福愉快的基础,又是事业成就的有力保证。

3. 自我激励　通过自我激励,满足事业上的成就欲,是成年人心理活动的主流。个人生活幸福是事业成功之辅助,力争事业成就是人生意义所在。

二、身体护理

(一)保证睡眠

首先养成良好的作息习惯,营造好的睡眠环境。养成按时入睡和起床的良好习惯,稳定睡眠,避免引起大脑皮质细胞的过度疲劳;卧房内的温度适中,房内使用一些温和的色彩搭配,这样可以使心情放松,适宜睡眠。精神放松疏解压力:缓解自身的压力,如通过睡前的适量运动、听音乐、头部按摩来疏解压力。睡前短距离的散步;睡觉时播放小夜曲等轻柔、舒缓的乐曲;使用按摩疗法,在入睡前按摩头部、面部、耳后、脖子等部位,都可以缓解全身的疲劳,促进睡眠。

(二)健康饮食

日常食物摄入以谷类作物为主,蛋、肉、豆类比较丰富。成年期男性蔬菜、水果、乳类摄入量偏少;女性豆类、鱼虾类摄入量较低。从能量来源上看,脂肪占有很大比重。因大量摄入脂肪,使得成年人过早出现高血压、冠心病等疾病。除此以外,成年人的水果、蔬菜摄入量低,导致体内维生素、矿物质缺乏,严重影响新陈代谢。因而在食物的选择上,应包含谷类、肉类、乳类、蔬菜、水果。平时要注意食物的搭配以保证其营养均衡。

(三)运动锻炼

每天坚持运动,有助于缓解工作疲劳,提高抵抗力,活动关节,加速身体新陈代谢,促进血液循环,预防"三高"(高血压、高血脂、高血糖),十分有益于身体健康。

有氧运动是成年人最常见、最有效的运动方式。在进行中等强度有氧运动时,可将运动强度控制在60%～70%最大心率范围,或相当于主观体力感觉12～14级;在进行大强度有氧运动时,可将运动强度控制强度在70%～80%最大心率范围,或相当于主观体力感觉15～16级。成年人可采用以下3种方式进行有氧运动。①中等强度有氧运动:每周进行150 min以上的中等强度有氧运动:每天运动30 min或以上,每周运动5 d。②大强度有氧运动:每周进行75 min以上的大强度有氧运动。每天运动25 min或以上,每周运动3 d。③交替性有氧运动。每周交替进行中等强度、大强度有氧运动,如每周一、三、五进行30 min或以上的中等强度有氧运动,每周二、周日进行25 min或以上的大强度有氧运动。

对于身体状况好且有良好运动习惯的人,每周进行300 min中等强度有氧运动,或150 min大强度有氧运动,健身效果更明显。合理运动不仅可以增强体质,防治高血压、血脂异常、糖尿病等慢性疾病,而且可以有效地提高机体免疫力,对于预防乳腺癌、结肠癌等癌症也有积极作用。对于控制或降低体重的成年人来讲,每天进行 60 min 有氧运动,可以控制体重的增加,每天进行 90 min 以上的有氧运动,可以减少体内脂肪含量,使体重下降,如果在运动的同时,配合控制饮食,降低体重效果更明显。

练习题

1. 埃里克森认为以下属于成年早期个体冲突的是(　　　)
　　A. 亲密对孤独　　　　　　B. 主动对内疚　　　　　　C. 勤奋对自卑　　　　　　D. 自我同一性对角色混乱

2. 中年期的年龄范围是(　　　)
　　A. 30 ~ 40 岁　　　　　　B. 35 ~ 40 岁　　　　　　C. 45 ~ 65 岁　　　　　　D. 50 ~ 65 岁

3. 女性更年期年龄在(　　　)
　　A. 30 ~ 40 岁　　　　　　B. 45 岁 ~ 55 岁　　　　　C. 60 ~ 65 岁　　　　　　D. 65 ~ 70 岁

4. 中年人的工作满意度(　　　)
　　A. 达到一生中的最低谷　　　　　　　　　　B. 达到一生中的最高峰
　　C. 和青年期相比没有什么特点　　　　　　　D. 起伏变化较大

5. 中年人对自我的看法(　　　)
　　A. 表现出消极的变化　　　　　　　　　　　B. 与青年期相比没有什么变化
　　C. 表现出更加积极的、满意的变化　　　　　D. 因人而异

参考答案

第九章　成年晚期个体的发展

▨▨▨▨▨ 学习目标 ▨▨▨▨▨

1. 掌握成年晚期面临的挑战、发展任务、主要的心理卫生问题及一般心理特点。
2. 熟悉成年晚期认知、情绪情感、个性和社会性发展变化的一般趋势或特点。
3. 了解合适老年人的活动,满足老年人需求。

成年晚期,亦称成人晚期、老年期,一般指从 65 岁到衰亡这段时期。成年晚期个体身心变化的基本特点是:尽管个别差异很大,但其总的趋势是逐渐表现出退行性变化。

第一节　成年晚期的认知特点

一、感知觉发生显著的退行性变化

(一)视觉减退

随着年老,眼睛晶状体弹性变小,调节力逐渐下降,因而时常看不清近物,出现老花眼。45 岁之前视力下降比较缓慢,一过 45 岁便加速下降。一般到 45 岁以后便需要戴老花眼镜。

(二)听觉减退

与视觉相比,老年人有听觉缺陷的为数更多。据统计,美国 65～74 岁的老年人中,听觉迟钝的占 13% ;75 岁以上的老年人中,26% 的有听觉缺陷。我国的调查发现,63.6% 的老年人听力减退,对高音的听力减退更明显,有些人听力减退到耳聋的程度。研究指出,人的听力最佳年龄是 20 岁,以后便缓慢下降。30 岁以后,听觉阈限随年龄增长而逐步提高。比斯利的研究指出,人一般超过 50 岁时听力就下降。研究者认为,50～59 岁可视为中国人听力老化的转折期。语言听觉理解力随年龄增长而逐渐下降,70～79 岁组开始明显下降,80～89 岁及 90 岁以上下降尤为明显。因此,与老年人讲话,关键部分要慢些,多重复几遍;同时,不要突然转换话题,要平视对象,这样,老年人就可以通过观察说话者的嘴唇活动判断话语。

(三)味觉减退

由于味道的感受器味蕾随着年龄的增长而减少,因而味觉的敏感性也随着年龄增长而下降。研究指出,人的味觉一般在 50 岁前无多大变化,而一过 50 岁,味觉的刺激阈限便增大。味觉的多样性也随年龄增长而减退,青年人能同时品尝出食品中的多种味道,而老年人往往只能感觉到其中的几种,他们对咸味的感知比对其他味道敏感些。

二、记忆随增龄而减退

在日常生活中，人们时常可以听到一些抱怨："我老了，记性坏了，经常丢三落四的。"人的记忆和年龄究竟是什么关系？人到老年期记忆真的衰退了吗？衰退的内部机制或原因是什么？

有心理学家根据有关记忆的实验研究，对记忆与年龄的关系做了这样的概括：儿童的记忆随年龄的增长而发展，到了成年期记忆达到最高峰。18～30岁是人的记忆的"黄金时期"，记忆的效率最高。35岁以后，记忆逐步减退。减退的趋势是：假定18～35岁时记忆的平均成绩为100%（最高），那么35～60岁时记忆的平均成绩则为95%，60～85岁时为80%～85%。我国的研究指出，人的记忆在40岁以后有一个较为明显的衰退阶段，然后维持在一个相对稳定的水平上，直到70岁以后又出现一个较明显的衰退阶段。可见就大多数老年人来说，其记忆变化的总趋势是随增龄而减退，主要表现为机械记忆减退，记忆广度变小，规定时间内的速度记忆能力下降，再认能力较差，回忆能力显著减退等。

三、思维的变化

一些心理学家关于思维的年龄差异的研究表明，人到老年期，概念学习、解决问题等思维过程的效能呈现出逐渐衰退的趋势。但由于思维是高级复杂的认识活动，这方面的研究进展缓慢，直到目前为止，人们对思维的衰退变化仍了解甚少，对许多问题仍存在着不同的观点。从现实生活来看，各国政府官员和大中型企业中的决策者主要是那些五六十岁甚至七十岁以上的中老年人，这表明他们仍具有较高的思维能力。可是实验室的研究结果表明，老年人解决问题的能力有普遍下降的趋势。至于何时开始下降，最后下降的幅度大小，研究的结论也多不一致。

第二节　成年晚期的情绪情感特点

成年晚期情绪情感的特点及影响因素既是发展心理学家关注的课题，也是关系到老年人心身健康和生活质量的现实问题。

一、比较容易产生消极的情绪情感

人到老年期，由于生理、心理的退行性变化以及退休后角色地位、社会交往的变化，比较容易产生抑郁感、孤独感、衰老感和自卑感等消极情绪情感。国内的某些调查资料说明了这一特点。上海的一项对164名退休老人的调查表明，有时有抑郁感（包括焦虑不安）的约占40%，有时有孤独感的占21.3%，经常有孤独感的占13.1%。北京的一项对53名离退休干部的调查指出，完全没有抑郁感的占42%，稍有和一般有抑郁感的分别占22%和34%，抑郁感较重者占2%；完全没有孤独感的占47%，稍有和一般有者各占23%；完全没有衰老感的占15%，稍有和一般有以及较重者分别占51%、30%和4%；老而不中用感的数据与此类似，稍有、一般有和较重者分别占53%、32%和2%。我们虽然不能仅根据这些初步调查对我国老年人目前的情绪情感做出结论，但这些调查结果起码给我们留下了这样的印象：我国老年人有各种消极情绪情感的占相当数量。

二、情感体验深刻而持久

老年人的情感体验比较深刻。这主要表现在他们的道德感方面。一个关于道德感的调查问卷中有一题要求对象对"你认为什么是最重要的基本道德?"进行选择,结果选择"热爱祖国"一项的百分率如下:18～30岁的占27.9%;31～45岁的占38.3%;46～60岁的占45.5%;60岁以上的占52.1%。可见,老年人把"热爱祖国"看成是最重要的基本道德的人数比例是各年龄组中最高的。在被问及"如果本市政府发布了一项新的有关人民生活的政策,你对此有不同意见,你会怎么办?"时,45岁以上两个年龄组(即中老组)中有接近半数的人选择"通过各种途径反映给政府部门",而45岁以下两个年龄组作此选择的人数则大大减少。在被问及"今后5年,我国政治环境将如何变化?"时,45岁以下的回答"不清楚"的百分率显著高于45岁以上的中年人。这说明我国大多数老年人对祖国、社会仍充满着政治热情,有高度的责任感。

第三节 成年晚期的护理工作

随着社会的进步和医疗技术的发达,我国人均寿命逐年提高,人口老龄化已成为医疗界乃至全社会共同面临的问题。对于医务人员来说,运用现有的医疗护理手段,尽最大可能地提高老年人的生活质量,是我们现阶段的重要任务。现将老年人常见健康问题及护理保健措施分析整理如下。

一、成年晚期常见健康问题

1. 退休不适综合征 老年人由于退休所致的社会地位、经济地位、生活环境等发生了改变,其活动空间和作息规律也随之发生改变,加上身体功能的衰退,尤其是听力和视力的减退,使他们无法与年轻人正常沟通与对话,这种巨大的落差常会导致出现身体和心理上的不适应,如空虚感、无用感、孤独感、被抛弃感等,导致部分老年人出现抑郁、自杀倾向。

2. 多种慢性病 随着生活条件的提高,生态环境的污染,不良的饮食习惯,不合理的饮食结构,老年人慢性病发病率逐年增多。目前,老年人最常患的慢性病有高血压、冠心病、糖尿病、脑卒中、恶性肿瘤、小脑退化综合征、帕金森病、慢性支气管炎等,这极大地影响了老年人的生活质量。

3. 空巢效应 子女长大后,因为种种原因,无法再与父母同住,又因为工作或学业繁忙,无法经常回家看望父母,与父母沟通越来越少。基于对儿女们的依恋和不舍,以及对儿女们在外的担忧,老人常常整日处于期盼、挂念、担心的负面情绪当中,这样极其不利于老年人健康。

二、成年晚期护理保健措施

1. 指导老年人自我保健 提高预防自理缺陷的意识:通过对老年人进行健康教育,使他们意识到自我照顾与帮助他人具有相同的社会价值,使他们自觉自愿地在生活上克服和预防自理缺陷。培养自我观察与判断能力:通过健康教育,使老年人通过看、听、闻、摸的方法了解自身的健康状况,一旦发现异常或疾病的早期症状,应及时到医院就医,主动寻求医务人员的帮助,以免延误诊断及治疗。

2. 创造良好居家环境 指导老年人创造舒适的生活环境:居室要光照充足;每日定时2～3次通风,通风时间以30 min左右为宜;室温适宜,夏季保持在26～28 ℃,冬季保持在20～22 ℃;湿度保持在50%左右;保持地面平坦、防滑。

3. 合理膳食 老年人的饮食原则是:①食物应粗细搭配,利于消化。②经常参加适当体力活动,以保持能量的平衡。此外,要防止老年人脱水,因为老年人渴觉不敏感,当感到口渴时已处于轻度脱水状态,因此,建议并督促老年人每日饮水不少于2 000 mL。

4.**保证良好的睡眠** 良好的睡眠能增强免疫力,使人精力充沛。因此,对于睡眠质量下降的老年人,应给与积极干预,措施如下。①生活要有规律,养成良好的生活习惯。②保持情绪稳定,做到劳逸结合。③创造适宜的睡眠环境:卧室光线柔和,睡前可听一些令人放松的轻音乐等。

5.**安全用药** 老年人大多患有多种慢性疾病,因此,需要长期反复用药,且多为联合用药。为老年人用药时应遵循科学的用药原则,尽可能降低用药的危险性,确保用药的安全和有效。因此,服药时应注意:①用药量不可过大。②用药种类不可过多。③严格遵照医嘱用药。④注意密切观察用药后的反应。⑤根据药品说明书储存和保管药物。见光易分解的药物,应避光保存,需低温保存的药物应放入恒温冰箱内,以免降低药效。

练习题

1.成年晚期一般是指( )
    A.50 岁以后   B.65 岁以后   C.70 岁以后   D.80 岁以后

2.老年期心理发展的总趋势是( )
    A.认知活动的退行性变化   B.人格出现偏差   C.情感脆弱   D.人际交往技能降低

3.老年期退行性变化出现最早的心理过程是( )
    A.感知觉   B.注意   C.记忆   D.思维

4.老年人的人格特征的重要变化是( )
    A.安全感增加   B.孤独感下降   C.适应性增加   D.拘泥刻板性

5.老年期人格的变化特点是( )
    A.安全感增加   B.孤独感降低   C.趋于激进   D.容易回忆往事

6.以下不属于老年丧失观认为老年期丧失的内容为( )
    A.心身健康   B.经济基础   C.情绪体验   D.生活价值

参考答案

■■■■■ 学习目标 ■■■■■

1.明确学习的概念。
2.理解早期学习理论。

第一节　学习的概念

一、学习过程

学习指由于先前的经验而发生的永久性行为变化。当一个人学习任何东西时,大脑的某些部分会发生变化,以记录他们学到的东西。

学习过程的模式见图10-1。

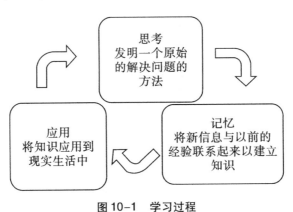

图 10-1　学习过程

二、新生儿的学习

新生儿除了控制眼睛和嘴巴外,几乎无法控制自己的肌肉。如果一个婴儿出生时可以完全控制所有肌肉,包括手臂、手、腿和脚,那会是一件好事吗?

在这样的情形之下,当父母不再夸耀他们发育超前的孩子后,他们会发现一件可怕的事情。一个行动不便但没有经验的婴儿会陷入所有可能的危险。从一开始,人类就需要了解什么是安全的,什么不是,我们可以去哪里,不应该去哪里。几乎我们所做的一切都需要不断学习和重新学习。

心理学家对学习进行了大量研究,在此过程中,他们开发和改进了研究方法,现在他们经常将其应用于其他心理调查领域。本章将讲解改变行为的过程——为什么你看到美味的食物时会舔嘴唇?为什么你会拒绝曾经让你生病的食物?为什么要小心处理锋利的刀具?为什么看到有人拿着刀向你冲过来,你会颤抖?

第二节　早期学习理论

一、经典条件反射

在 1900 年代初期,俄罗斯生理学家伊万·彼得罗维奇·巴甫洛夫因对消化的研究而获得诺贝尔生理学或医学奖,他偶然发现了一个可以为学习提供简单解释的观察结果。鉴于行为主义的兴起,巴甫洛夫提出想法的时机已经成熟。有一天,巴甫洛夫在进行消化研究时,注意到一只狗一看到经常喂它的实验室工作人员就会分泌消化液。因为这种分泌物明显取决于狗之前的经历,所以巴甫洛夫称之为"心理"分泌物。他获得了其他专家的帮助,他们发现用食物"逗弄"一只狗会产生唾液,这种唾液与任何反射一样可预测和自动产生。巴甫洛夫称其为条件反射,因为它取决于各种不同的条件。

例如,当食物在嘴里时就会分泌唾液。每当巴甫洛夫给狗食物时,狗就会流口水。食物与唾液的联系是自动的,不需要训练。巴甫洛夫称食物为非条件刺激,他称流口水为非条件反射。非条件刺激（UCS）是一种自动引发非条件反射的事件。非条件反射（UCR）是非条件刺激引起的动作。接下来巴甫洛夫引入了一种新的刺激——铃铛的声音。听到铃铛的声音,狗抬起耳朵环顾四周,但没有流口水,因此铃铛是对流口水的中性刺激。巴甫洛夫在给狗喂食前不久按下铃铛,将铃铛与食物配对几次后,狗一听到铃铛就开始流口水。

我们将铃铛称为条件刺激（CS）,因为狗对它的反应取决于前面的条件,即将条件刺激（CS）与非条件刺激（UCS）配对。伴随铃铛的流口水是条件反射（CR）。条件反射（CR）是条件刺激（CS）由于条件反射（训练）过程而引起的任何反应。一开始,条件刺激（CS）不会引起明显的反应,在反复刺激之后,它会引发条件反射（CR）（图 10-2）。

（一）其他经典条件反射举例

在牙钻对你的牙齿造成不愉快的体验之前,你会听到牙钻的声音。在经历这些以后,牙钻的声音会引起你的焦虑。

非条件刺激＝钻孔→非条件反射＝紧张

条件刺激＝牙钻的声音→条件反射＝紧张

哺乳母亲通过将婴儿放在她的乳房上来回应婴儿的哭声,从而刺激乳汁的流动。经过几天的重复,婴儿的哭声足以让乳汁开始流动。

非条件刺激＝婴儿吸吮→非条件反射＝乳汁流动

条件刺激＝婴儿的哭声→条件反射＝乳汁流动

（二）经典条件反射的附加现象

建立或加强条件反射的过程称为习得。在发现经典条件反射后,巴甫洛夫和其他学者改变了实验程序以产生其他结果。以下是一些主要现象。

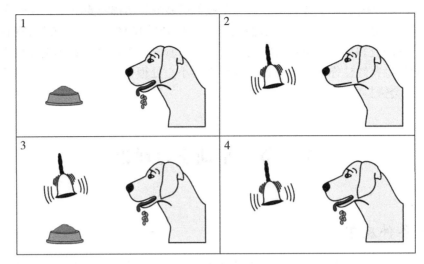

图 10-2　经典条件反射

1. 消退　假设有人用蜂鸣器发出蜂鸣声,然后向你的眼睛吹了一口空气。重复几次后,你一听到蜂鸣声就开始闭上眼睛。现在蜂鸣器在没有吹气的情况下反复响起,你会做出什么反应?

你第一次会眨眼,也许还有第二次和第三次,但没多久,你就停下了。这种条件反射的降低称为消退。为了消除经典的条件反射,重复呈现条件刺激(CS)而没有非条件刺激(UCS)。也就是说,当条件刺激预测非条件刺激时发生条件反射(CR)的获取,而当条件刺激不再预测非条件刺激时发生消退。

消退不等于遗忘。两者都削弱了习得的反应,但它们以不同的方式出现。在没有提醒或练习的情况下,你会在很长一段时间内忘记。消退是由于一种特定的体验而发生的——在没有非条件刺激的情况下感知条件刺激。如果习得是学会做出反应,那么消退就是学会抑制它。

不要被消退一词的含义所误导。在动物或植物物种消退后,它就永远消失了。在经典条件反射中,消退并不意味着消失。消退会抑制反应。可以把它想象成灭火:在大火上浇水可以扑灭大火,但一些焖烧的余烬可能会徘徊很久,并且很容易重新点燃大火。

2. 自发恢复　假设你正在进行经典条件反射试验。起初,你会反复听到蜂鸣器(CS)的声音,然后向你的眼睛吹气(UCS),然后蜂鸣器停止伴随吹气。几次试验后,你对蜂鸣器的反应消失了。接下来,你等待一段时间,什么也没有发生,直到突然你再次听到蜂鸣器。你会怎么做?很可能,你至少会稍微眨一下眼睛。自发恢复是在延迟后暂时恢复消失的反射。

为什么会出现自发恢复?可以这样想:起初,蜂鸣器预测到你的眼睛前会吹出一股空气,然后它消失了。你的反应更容易受到最近的刺激的影响。几个小时后,两种体验相对来说没有哪一个明显靠近现在了,所以这两种获得和消退的影响作用几乎相同。

二、操作性条件反射

假设另一个国家的家庭在你出生时收养了你。之后你生活在一个有着不同语言、习俗、食物、宗教等的土地上。毫无疑问,你会在很多方面有所不同。但是那个替代的"你"和现在的"你"有什么共同之处吗?还是你的文化和环境完全塑造了你的行为?环境决定论最极端的说法来自行为主义的创始人之一约翰·沃森。他说,给我十几个健康的婴儿,发育良好,让我在自己指定的世界抚养他们,我保证随机挑选其中的任何一个,都能训练他成为我可能选择的任何类型的专家——医生、律师、艺术家、商人、领袖,甚至是乞丐、小偷,无论他的祖先的天赋、嗜好、倾向、能力、职业和种族如何。

当然,沃森从来没有机会证明他的观点。没有人能够给他一个孩子和他自己指定的世界。如果他或其他人真的能够完全控制环境,是否有可能控制孩子最终的命运?毕竟,我们可能永远不会知道,因为道德的制约存在于这个世界。尽管如此,研究学习的研究人员的目标之一是了解环境变化会导致什么样的行为变化。操作性条件反射是由斯金纳提出的,他认为,一个人因正确反应而获得奖励,而不因错误反应而获得奖励的学习方式,使我们将一种反应和其后果关联。

操作性行为作用于环境产生强化,并因强化而更加强化。

例如:斯金纳的涉及老鼠、盒子和食物的实验。

任何行为研究人员面临的一个问题是如何定义反应。想象一下观察孩子并试图记录"攻击性行为"。什么是攻击性行为?什么不是?斯金纳通过简化情况进行了测量:他设置了一个盒子,称为"操作性调节室"(或"斯金纳盒子"),老鼠在其中按下杠杆或鸽子啄一个发光的"钥匙"来接收食物。他在操作上将反应定义为动物按下杠杆或"钥匙"所做的任何事情。因此,如果老鼠用鼻子而不是爪子按压杠杆,反应仍然有效。如果鸽子用它的翅膀敲击"钥匙"而不是用它的喙啄它,仍然算数。行为是由它的结果来定义的,而不是由肌肉运动来定义的(图 10-3)。

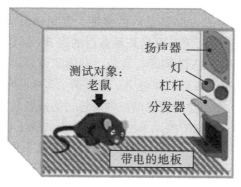

图 10-3 斯金纳盒子

令人愉快的结果会增加行为重复的机会,不愉快的后果会减少重复行为的机会,这是在一种称为行为矫正的治疗形式中使用的方法(表 10-1)。

表 10-1 斯金纳盒子实验说明

	给老鼠的东西	从老鼠身上拿走的东西
增加重复行为的可能性	积极的巩固 当杠杆被按下老鼠获得食物(在绿灯亮起后)	消极的巩固 当杠杆被按下的时候大的声响停止
	积极的惩罚 当杠杆被按下(在红灯亮起后)老鼠被电击	消极的惩罚 在此情景中不可用

1. 强化与惩罚 有些事件对强化某些人的行为来说非常有效,而对另一些人则不然。有的人会仅仅为了得高分而玩电子游戏很多小时。在一个古怪的实验中,母鼠可以按下杠杆将更多的小老鼠送进笼子。它们不断地按,增加越来越多的幼鼠。关于什么是好的强化刺激,什么不是,有什么固定的模式吗?

我们可能会猜测强化刺激对个体在生物学上是有用的,但很多不是。例如,糖精是一种甜的物质,但在生物学上是无用的化学物质。它可以作为强化刺激。对许多人来说,酒精和烟草比富含维生素的蔬菜更能作为强化剂。所以生物学上的有用性并不能定义强化。

定义强化的一种有用方法依赖于平衡的概念。如果你可以随心所欲地度过一天,你会如何分配时间?假设你一天中30%的时间在睡觉,10%的时间在吃饭,8%的时间在锻炼,11%的时间在阅读,9%的时间与朋友交谈,2%的美容时间,2%的时间弹钢琴,等等。现在假设有什么东西让你在一两天内远离这些活动之一,根据强化的不平衡原理,任何阻止活动的东西都会产生不平衡,进行该活动的机会将使你恢复平衡,而恢复平衡的机会就是强化。

当然,有些活动比其他活动更加重要。如果你被剥夺了氧气,那么呼吸的机会会非常具有强化作用。如果你被剥夺了阅读时间或电话时间,强化值就少了。

2. 初级和次级强化刺激　心理学家区分由于自身特性而增强的初级强化刺激(或非条件性强化刺激)和通过与其他事物关联而增强的次级强化刺激(或条件性强化刺激)。食物和水是主要的强化刺激。金钱(次级强化刺激)之所以成为强化刺激,是因为我们可以用它来换取食物或其他主要强化刺激。一个学生知道一个好成绩会赢得认可,一个员工知道提高生产力会赢得雇主的称赞。我们大部分时间都在为次级强化刺激工作。

3. 惩罚　与强化刺激相比,惩罚会降低反应的概率。强化刺激可以是某物的呈现(例如,接受食物)或移除(例如,止痛)。同样,惩罚可以是某种东西的表现(例如,接受疼痛)或移除(例如,拒绝食物)。当惩罚快速且可预测时,惩罚是最有效的。不确定或延迟的惩罚效果较差。例如,你因触摸火炉而感到的灼伤可以非常有效地教你避免一些事情。多年后吸烟可能使你患上癌症的威胁也可能有效,但效果较差。惩罚并不总是有效的。如果惩罚的威胁总是有效的,犯罪率将为零。

斯金纳在一项著名的实验室研究中测试了惩罚。他首先训练了食物匮乏的老鼠按杠杆来获取食物,然后他停止给予它们食物。在最初的 10 min 内,一些老鼠不仅没有得到食物,而且每按一次杠杆,它们的爪子就会被打一下。被惩罚的老鼠暂时抑制了它们的按压,但从长远来看,它们的按压次数与未受到惩罚的老鼠一样多。斯金纳得出结论,惩罚不会产生长期影响。

然而,这个结论是夸大其词的。更好的结论是,当没有其他反应可用时,惩罚不会大大削弱反应,因为斯金纳的饥饿老鼠没有其他方法来寻找食物(如果有人因为呼吸而惩罚你,你仍然会继续呼吸)。

尽管如此,替代惩罚的方法通常更有效。我们怎样才能让司机遵守学区限速?警告他们罚款不是很有效。即使在该地区派驻警察也取得了有限的成功。一个令人惊讶的有效方式是张贴驾驶员反馈标志,该标志张贴速度限制和基于雷达传感器的"您的速度"公告。仅仅获得个人反馈就可以提高驾驶员对法律的认识和遵守法律的可能性。

对孩子进行体罚,例如打屁股,是好主意还是坏主意?打屁股在许多国家都是非法的,主要是在欧洲。许多心理学家强烈反对打屁股,建议父母简单地与孩子推理或使用非物理的管教方法,例如暂停或失去看电视权利或其他特权。有什么证据支持这一建议?所有研究都提出了体罚与行为问题之间的相关性。经常被打屁股的孩子往往行为不端。你应该看到解释这个结果的问题:这可能意味着打屁股会导致行为不端,或者可能意味着行为不端的孩子会激怒他们的父母打他们。这也可能意味着在压力大的家庭、父母冲突频繁的家庭或有其他可能导致不当行为的因素的家庭中,打屁股更为常见。一种更好的研究将经常被打屁股的孩子与经常受到非体罚的惩罚方式的来自相似背景的孩子进行比较。这类研究表明,被打屁股的人和受到其他类型惩罚的人之间没有区别。因此,似乎不当行为导致的惩罚(无论何种类型)比惩罚导致的不当行为更多。

对于类似于虐待儿童的严厉惩罚,结论是不同的。可能的结果包括反社会行为、自卑和对父母的敌意,以及终生健康问题的风险增加。

我们可以通过表 10-2 的总结比较经典条件反射和操作性条件反射。

表 10-2　比较经典条件反射和操作性条件反射

项目	经典条件反射	操作性条件反射
反射	不自愿的,自动的	自愿的,操作环境
获得	与事件关联,条件性刺激联系非条件刺激	反应与一种后果关联(强化刺激或惩罚)
消退	条件反射下降:当条件刺激单独重复	反应减弱:当强化刺激停止
认知过程	实验对象发展出条件刺激预示着非条件刺激到达的期望	实验对象发展出一种反应会被强化或者惩罚的期望;同时展示出潜在的学习,即使没有了强化刺激
生理倾向	自然倾向限制了哪些刺激和反应可以很容易地联系起来	实验对象能更好地学习与其自然行为相似的行为;不自然的行为本能地回到自然的行为

三、社会学习理论

社会学习理论是基于阿尔弗雷德班杜拉的工作。它也被称为社会认知理论(SCT)。该理论试图理解和解释我们如何相互学习所涉及的过程。它侧重于通过观察、模仿和建模进行的学习。

它为理解、预测和潜在改变人类行为提供了一个框架。

正如许多鸟类从其他鸟类那里学习它们的歌声一样,人类显然也从彼此身上学到了很多东西。想想所有你没有通过反复试验学到的东西:你不会随便穿衣服,等着看哪件衣服能带来最好的效果,相反,你学习其他人穿着的款式;如果你在做饭,你也不会随便编食谱,你从其他人的推荐开始;如果你在跳舞,你不会随意尝试每一个可能的肌肉运动,你会复制别人的动作。

根据社会学习理论,我们通过观察他人的行为来了解许多行为。例如,如果你想学习驾驶汽车,你首先要观察已经熟练的人。当你尝试开车时,你会因为驾驶而受到强化和惩罚(可能是受伤),如果你驾驶水平不好,但你对他人的观察有助于你的进步。

社会学习是一种操作性条件反射,其基本机制是相似的。但是,社交信息通常比尝试自己从头开始学习更快、更有效。行为、个人因素和环境因素在学习过程中都发挥着重要作用。它们不断地相互影响。

班杜拉的理论认为,孩子通过观察他人来学习;同一组刺激可能会引起不同人或同一人在不同时间的不同反应;环境与人的行为是相互关联的;性格是 3 个因素相互作用的结果:环境、行为和一个人的心理过程。

班杜拉的“波波”娃娃实验:阿尔伯特班杜拉研究了模仿对学习攻击行为的作用。他们让一组孩子观看成人或卡通人物猛烈攻击充气“波波”娃娃的短片,另一组观看了不同的短片。然后他们把孩子们留在了一个有“波波”娃娃的房间里。只有看过攻击娃娃的短片的孩子会攻击娃娃,使用许多他们刚刚看到的相同动作。这意味着,孩子们会复制他们在他人身上看到的攻击性行为。

练习题

1. 下列属于学习现象的是( )
   A. 老鼠打洞 B. 吃酸的东西会流唾液
   C. 儿童模仿电影中的人物 D. 蜘蛛织网

2. 根据经典条件反射作用理论,铃声可以诱发狗的唾液分泌反应,则铃声是( )
   A. 条件刺激 B. 非条件刺激 C. 条件反射 D. 非条件反射

3. 学习会影响我们的大脑,属于一种( )
   A. 心理变化 B. 物理变化 C. 感知变化 D. 化学变化

4. 在哺乳活动中,母亲一听到孩子的哭声就开始分泌乳汁,这属于( )
   A. 非条件反射 B. 条件反射 C. 动作技能 D. 态度

5. 经常去医院治疗牙齿的人听到牙钻的声音就会紧张,这属于( )
   A. 非条件反射 B. 条件反射 C. 动作技能 D. 态度

6. 在巴甫洛夫的经典实验中,如果在条件反射建立以后,反复响铃却不提供食物,狗的唾液分泌现象会消失,这属于( )
   A. 消退 B. 自发恢复 C. 刺激泛化 D. 刺激分化

7. 当学生取得好的成绩后,老师和家长给予表扬和鼓励,学生会更喜欢学习。所以表扬和鼓励是( )
   A. 正强化 B. 负强化 C. 条件刺激 D. 非条件刺激

8. 看见路上的垃圾后绕道走开,这种行为是( )
   A. 强化 B. 惩罚 C. 逃避条件作用 D. 消退

9. 行为塑造和行为矫正的原理和依据是( )
   A. 操作性条件作用理论 B. 经典条件作用理论 C. 精神分析理论 D. 认知理论

10. 由于一个学生进步明显,老师取消了对他的处分,这属于( )
    A. 正强化 B. 负强化 C. 奖励 D. 惩罚

参考答案

第十一章　智　力

===== 学习目标 =====

1.掌握智力的概念。
2.熟悉智力的研究任务。
3.了解智力的相关理论。

第一节　智力的概述

什么是智力？不同的学者对此有不同的认识。皮亚杰认为，智慧的本质从生物学来说是一种适应，是同化和顺应之间的一种特殊的能力。韦克斯勒将智力定义为"智力是个人行动有目的、思维合理、应付环境有效的一种聚集的或全面的才能。"所以说聚集，是因为它由诸要素或诸能力所构成；所以说全面，是因为人类行为是以整体为特征。

一、智力理论

爱德华·李·桑代克(1874—1949)，美国心理学家，1912年当选为美国心理学会主席，1917年当选为国家科学院院士。桑代克提出了"智力三因论"，他认为可能有抽象智力(包括心智能力，特别是处理语言和数学符号的能力)、具体智力(一个人处理事物的能力)、社会智力(人与人相互交往的能力)3种智力，并且认为这3种智力是由遗传、环境和教育3个因素共同作用的。

1.抽象智力　包括心智能力，特别是处理语言和数学符号的能力。一个具有抽象智力的人能够发现要解决的符号之间的关系问题。例如：医生、律师和数学家。

2.具体智力　即一个人处理事物的能力。例如：机械工程师和受过训练的工业工程师工人们有大量的机械设备智力。

3.社会智力　即处理人与人之间相互交往的能力。例如：推销员、外交官和政治家要善于交际。

二、多元智能理论

霍华德·加德纳，是世界著名教育心理学家，最为人知的成就是提出"多元智能理论"，被誉为"多元智能理论"之父。

加德纳认为，支撑多元智能理论的是个体身上相对独立存在着的、与特定的认知领域和知识领域相联系的8种智能：语言智能、节奏智能、数理智能、空间智能、动觉智能、自省智能、交流智能和自然观察智能。

多元智能理论认为,智能是在某种社会或文化环境的价值标准下,个体用以解决自己遇到的真正难题或生产及创造出有效产品所需要的能力。具体包含如下含义。

1.每一个体的智能各具特点 根据加德纳的多元智能理论,作为个体,我们每个人都同时拥有相对独立的8种智能,但每个人身上的8种相对独立的智能在现实生活中并不是绝对孤立、毫不相干的,而是以不同方式、不同程度有机地组合在一起。正是这8种智能在每个人身上以不同方式、不同程度组合,使得每一个人的智能各具特点。

2.个体智能的发展方向和程度受环境和教育的影响和制约 在多元智能理论看来,个体智能的发展受到环境包括社会环境、自然环境和教育条件的极大影响与制约,其发展方向和程度因环境和教育条件不同而表现出差异。尽管各种环境和教育条件下的人们身上都存在着8种智能,但不同环境和教育条件下人们智能的发展方向和程度有着明显的区别。

3.智能强调的是个体解决实际问题的能力和生产及创造出社会需要的有效产品的能力 在加德纳的多元智能理论看来,智能应该强调两个方面的能力,一个方面的能力是解决实际问题的能力,另一个方面的能力是生产及创造出社会需要的有效产品的能力。根据加德纳的分析,传统的智能理论产生于重视言语-语言智能和逻辑-数理智能的现代工业社会,智能被解释为一种以语言能力和数理逻辑能力为核心的整合的能力。

4.多元智能理论重视的是多维地看待智能问题的视角 在加德纳看来,承认智能是由同样重要的多种能力而不是由一两种核心能力构成,承认各种智能是多维度地、相对独立地表现出来而不是以整合的方式表现出来,应该是多元智能理论的本质之所在。

第二节 智力和智商

智商就是智力商数。智力通常叫智慧,也叫智能。智力是人们认识客观事物并运用知识解决实际问题的能力。智力包括多个方面,如观察力、记忆力、想象力、分析判断能力、思维能力、应变能力等。智力的高低通常用智力商数来表示,用以标示智力发展水平。

(一)智力测验

智力测验是有关人的普通心智功能的各种测验的总称,又称普通能力测验。智力测验的作用是诊断、收集基础数据、评估心理残疾、评估治疗。现在常用测验包括:比奈-西蒙智力量表、韦克斯勒智力量表、斯坦福-比奈智力量表、瑞文标准智力测验、军队甲种团体智力测验和军队乙种团体智力测验。

1905年,法国心理学家比奈·阿尔弗雷德(Binet Alfred,1857—1911)和他的学生编制了世界上第一套智力量表,根据这套智力量表将一般人的平均智商定为100。1916年,特曼教授把这套量表介绍到美国并修订为斯坦福-比奈智力量表,并用心理年龄与生理年龄之比作为评定儿童智力水平的指数,这个比被称为智商(IQ),用公式表示即是:IQ=MA(心理年龄)/CA(生理年龄)×100。在当代测试中,平均水平给定年龄的表现分数为100分。人们称这种智商为比率智商。

(二)其他测试

1.能力倾向测试 也称能力测试,是指测试受测者的较稳定的、表现在认知能力方面的心理特质,主要体现人在外部环境影响下,较不易改变的那些认知特点,如人的观察力、注意力、记忆力、理解力、抽象思维能力、判断推理能力等,在挑选企业经营管理者时常用到这种形式。

2.成就测验 或称成绩测验,主要考察受测者在学习和训练后所具有的知识和技能水平。由于它被广泛地应用在教育工作中,因此,有时也被称为教育测试(educational test)。根据不同的标准,还可以对之进行更为细致的分类。影响成就测验成绩的不仅是能力,而且包括通过学习所掌握的知识。

(三)影响智力的因素

1.遗传　与智商相关的基因在不同人种中有不同频率的分布,平均智商高的人种的智商基因比平均智商低的人种多。一般说父母智商高,孩子的智商也不会低。这种遗传因素还表现在血缘关系上,父母同是本地人,孩子平均智商为102;而隔省结婚的父母所生的孩子智商达109;父母是表亲,低智商的孩子明显增加。

2.精神残疾　21-三体综合征(唐氏综合征)、孤独症等。例如21-三体综合征,患儿在出生时即已有明显的特殊面容,且常呈现嗜睡和喂养困难,其智能低下表现随年龄增长而逐渐明显,智商25~50,动作发育和性发育都延迟。患儿眼距宽,鼻根低平,眼裂小,眼外侧上斜、有内眦赘皮,外耳小,舌胖、常伸出口外,流涎多,身材矮小,头围小于正常,头前后径短,枕部平呈扁头,颈短,皮肤宽松,骨龄常落后于年龄,出牙延迟且常错位,头发细软而较少、发旋多居中,前囟闭合晚,顶枕中线可有第三囟门,四肢短,由于韧带松弛,关节可过度弯曲,手指粗短,小指中节骨发育不良使小指向内弯曲,指骨短,手掌三叉点向远端移位,常见通贯掌纹、草鞋足,拇趾球部约半数患儿呈弓形皮纹。

患儿常伴有先天性心脏病等其他畸形,因免疫功能低下,易患各种感染,白血病的发生率比一般儿童增高10~30倍,如存活至成人期,则常在30岁以后即出现阿尔茨海默病症状。

3.母乳　母乳中含有多种促进儿童智力发育的活性物质,特别是对智力发育有重要影响的牛磺酸比牛奶要高出10倍之多。据调查,吃母乳长大的儿童比吃代乳品长大的儿童智商要高出3~10分。

4.饮食　饮食单调导致某些微量元素不足,或者饮食量过少,蛋白质等营养严重缺乏的情况下会导致智力发育受阻。摄入过多重金属元素如铅、铜等也会影响智力。

5.体重　体重超过正常儿童20%的孩子,其视觉、听力、接受知识的能力都会处于较低的水平。这是因为肥胖儿过多的脂肪进入脑内,妨碍神经细胞的发育和神经纤维增生。

6.环境　生活在枯燥环境里的儿童,如弃婴,得不到母爱及良好的教育,智商会较低。据研究调查表明,这类孩子3岁时平均智商仅为60.5;反之,处于良好环境的3岁儿童智商平均为91.8。

7.药物　某些药物会影响儿童的智力,如长期服用抗癫痫药物可使智商偏低,当停药若干年后,智商便会有所提高。

第三节　情　商

情商,通常是指情绪商数,它是近年来心理学家们提出的与智商相对应的概念。从简单的层次上下定义,提高情商的基础是培养自我意识,从而增强理解自己及表达自己的能力。

戈尔曼和其他研究者认为,情商由自知、自控、自励、通情达理和和谐相处这5种特征组成。

1.自知　就是能准确地识别、评价自己和他人的情绪,能及时察觉自己的情绪变化,能归结情绪产生的原因。

2.自控　就是适应性地调节、引导、控制、改善自己和他人的情绪,能够使自己摆脱强烈的焦虑、忧郁,能积极应对危机,并能增进实现目标的情绪力量。自控包括自我监督、自我管理、自我疏导、自我约束和尊重现实。尊重现实包括尊重自己的现实、他人的现实和周围环境的现实。

3. **自励** 就是利用情绪信息,整顿情绪,增强注意力,调动自己的精力和活力,适应性地确立目标,创造性地实现目标。自励就是有上进心、进取心,确立奋斗目标,并为之而积极努力。

4. **通情达理** 就是能设身处地考虑他人的情绪感受和行为原因,具备换位思考的能力和习惯,理解和认可情绪差别,能和与自己的观念不一致的人和平相处,理解别人的感受,察觉别人的真正需要,具有同情心。

5. **和谐相处** 就是能妥善处理人际问题,与他人和谐相处。在专业分工越来越细的前提下,相互协作变得越来越重要,时代呼唤团队合作精神,时代需要人人相互信赖、相互尊重和相互协作。协作的作用在于提高组织的绩效,使团队的工作业绩超过成员个体业绩的简单之和,从而形成强大的团队凝聚力和整体战斗力,最终实现团队目标。只有真正融入了团队,才能保证工作的效率和质量。

练习题

1. 试比较下列 4 个儿童的智商,智商最高的是( )
   A. 实足年龄 5 岁智力年龄 6 岁   B. 实足年龄 6 岁智力年龄 7 岁
   C. 实足年龄 5 岁智力年龄 8 岁   D. 实足年龄 7 岁智力年龄 8 岁

2. 所谓智力,主要是指( )
   A. 能力   B. 一般能力   C. 特殊能力   D. 观察能力

3. 编制第一个正式智力测验量表的是( )
   A. 吉尔福特   B. 韦克斯勒   C. 比奈西蒙   D. 推孟

4. 观察力、记忆力、思维力等均属于( )
   A. 特殊能力   B. 一般能力   C. 鉴别力   D. 操作能力

5. 测量智商的正确公式是( )
   A. $MA/CA \times 100$ B. $CA/MA \times 100$ C. $MA-CA$ D. CA/MA

6. 仿效他人的言行举止而引起的与之相类似的行为活动的能力是( )
   A. 模仿能力   B. 操作能力   C. 创造能力   D. 认知能力

7. 产生新思想、发现和创造新事物的能力被称为( )
   A. 创造能力   B. 操作能力   C. 模仿能力   D. 认知能力

8. 为表示一个儿童的智力水平,提出智力商数的概念,简称智商,缩写为( )
   A. EQ   B. MQ   C. IQ   D. CQ

9. 美国心理学家韦克斯勒依据统计学原理提出了智商的新的计算法,称为( )
   A. 相对智商   B. 绝对智商   C. 比率智商   D. 离差智商

10. 在智力发展水平上,人类的智力分布曲线基本上呈现的形态是( )
    A. 两头小   B. 中间大   C. 正态分布   D. 偏态分布

参考答案

第十二章　动　机

1. 掌握动机的概念。
2. 熟悉动机的分类与相关理论。
3. 了解动机在临床护理中的应用。

第一节　动机的概述

动机指的是作用于我们自身或内在的力量,它能启动、维持和指导我们的行为。它是一种内部的心理过程,是个人内在的需求、欲望、愿望或动力,激励人们采取行动以实现目标的过程。动机不能被直接观察到,但我们可以通过个体对任务的选择、努力的程度、对活动的坚持性以及言语表达等外部表现间接推断动机。

一、动机行为

动机引导并激活行为,直到实现目标,由动机引导的行为都有明确的目标。动机行为因人而异,视情况而定。相同的动机,不同的个体可以表现出不同的行为;相同的动机,同一个体在不同的时候也可以表现出不同的行为;同样的行为,也可能是由不同的动机引起的。动机行为受很多方面的影响,主要包括内在需要和外在诱因。动机就是导致我们在特定时间以特定方式行动的各种生理和心理因素。

二、动机模型

许多有动机的活动开始于一种需要或内在的缺乏或缺陷,这种需求导致人们产生动力(一种充满活力的激励状态),去达成期望的目标,一旦目标实现,就会让人产生满足感,这种满足感又会反馈给最初的需求或期望(图12-1)。动机就是个体为达到一个目标(动机行为的目标)而设计的驱动激活反应(一个或一系列的行动)。

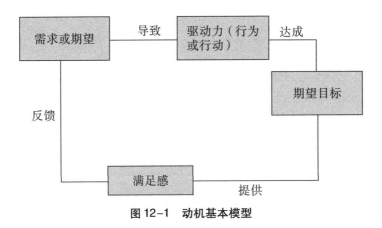

图 12-1　动机基本模型

第二节　动机的分类与相关理论

一、动机的分类

动机可以分为三大类:原始动机、刺激动机、次要动机。

(一)原始动机

最重要的原始动机包括饥饿、口渴、避免疼痛、呼吸、睡眠、排泄和调节体温等,它是维持生命所必须满足的动机。这里主要介绍一下饥饿动机。

饥饿是由于体内缺乏食物或营养而引起的一种生理不平衡状态,它表现为一定程度的紧张不安,甚至是某种折磨和痛苦,从而形成个体内在的压力,并驱使个体产生进食活动。饥饿感与很多因素相关。首先,饥饿感与胃部收缩有关,但胃部收缩不是产生饥饿感的必要条件。许多人的胃被切除后,仍能感到饥饿,并照常进食。其次,饥饿感与体内血糖水平高低相关。如果血糖水平下降,饥饿感就会增加,但胰岛素与血糖并不是调节饥饿感唯一的化学物质。再者,饥饿的产生还与中枢神经系统的某些部位的功能有关,在动物的下丘脑中就发现了所谓的“饥饿中枢”和“厌食中枢”。“饥饿中枢”会分泌一种引发饥饿的激素——促食欲素,当给老鼠注射这种激素时,它们会变得狼吞虎咽。而当“厌食中枢”受到刺激时,动物将停止进食。

(二)刺激动机

刺激动机包括活动、兴趣、探索、操纵(抱、触摸)和接触(亲近、情感)等,是个体对刺激、信息或知识的需求。这些动机推动人们积极地探寻外界世界。这里重点介绍兴趣。

兴趣是人们探究某种事物或从事某种活动的心理倾向,它以认识或探索外界的需要为基础,是推动人们认识事物、探求真理的重要动机。当兴趣指向某种活动时,这种动机叫爱好。人们对自己感兴趣的事物或活动会表现出巨大的积极性和关注度。婴儿出生后,对环境中出现的新奇事物产生的惊奇和兴奋的反应,就是个体对环境的一种探究活动。

(三)次要动机

许多次要动机都与对权力、从属关系(与他人在一起的需要)、认可、地位、安全和成就的习得需求有关,它推动个体主动与他人交往,希望获得社会与他人的赞许,希望参与某种社会团体,并能在其中获得某种地位。这是基于学习的需要、动力和目标之上的动机,例如金钱对婴儿来说毫无价值,正是通过学习,金钱才变得有价值,成为行为的动力。接下来,重点介绍权利动机。

权力动机是指人们具有的某种支配和影响他人以及周围环境的内在驱力。在权力动机的支配下,人们在活动中会积极参与和奉献,并有成为领导者的愿望。按个体行为的目标来分,权力动机可以分为个人化权力动机和社会化权力动机。具有个人化权力动机的个体寻求权力是为了满足个人的私欲或利益。具有社会化权力动机的个体寻求权力是为了他人,在行为上表现为关心社会、关心他人,以个人的知识、观念等方式影响他人。

二、人本主义理论

人本主义理论的代表人物是亚伯拉罕·马斯洛和卡尔·罗杰斯。人本主义心理学认为人的本质是好的、善良的,人有自由意志,有自我实现的需要。

(一)马斯洛需要层次理论

马斯洛提出需要层次理论,他认为人的需要是有5个等级构成的(图12-2)。

1. 生理需要　人们对食物、水分、空气、排泄、睡眠、性等的需要。他们在人的所有需要中是最重要的,也是最有力量的。

2. 安全需要　人们对稳定、安全、受到保护、有秩序,能免除恐惧、焦虑和混乱的折磨等的需要。如果生理需要相对充分地得到了满足后,就会出现安全需要。

3. 归属需要　人们对与其他人建立联系,如结交朋友、追求爱情、参加一个团体并在其中获得某种地位等的需要。如果生理需要和安全需要都得到很好的满足,归属需要就会产生。

4. 尊重需要　它包括自尊和希望受到别人的尊重。尊重需要的满足会使个体相信自己的价值,使个体更有能力,更富有创造性。相反,自尊缺乏的个体会自卑,缺乏信心。

5. 自我实现需要　它表现为人们追求实现自己能力或潜能的最大发展。自我实现的途径是因人而异的。自我实现需要是最高层次的需要,它的产生有赖于前述4种需要的满足。

马斯洛认为这5种需要都是人的基本需要,它们是与生俱来的,按高低构成了不同的等级,激励和指引着个体的行为,并且需要的层次越低,力量就越强大,层次越高,力量相对较弱。只有低级需要得到满足或部分满足时,才有可能出现更高一级的需要。当然,也有例外,有人为了满足高级需要可以牺牲低级需要,比如有些人为实现心中的信念与理想甘愿牺牲性命。

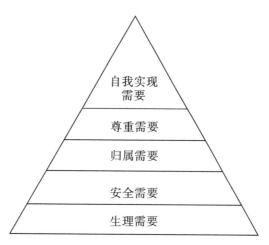

图12-2　马斯洛需要层次理论

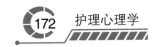
（二）马斯洛的动机类型

马斯洛把动机分为两种类型：内在动机和外在动机。

1. 内在动机　动机来源于内在驱力，是个体内在需要激发的动机，个体所做出于个人兴趣、挑战、享受。

2. 外在动机　动机来自外部驱动因素，是个体在外界的要求与外力的作用下所产生的行为动机，个体所做源于人以外的因素，如奖励、有形收益等。

第三节　临床护理中的应用

一、需要在临床护理中的应用

在临床护理工作中，患者因为病种、病情严重程度、文化程度、职业、经济条件和个性特征等的不同，在临床表现中表现出的需要特点也各不相同。护士应了解满足基本需求的必要性，尽可能满足患者的合理需要，例如患者对适当食物、水或液体、空气或氧气的需要，理解患者追求生命安全、健康安全时出现的各种心理感受，从而进行针对性的护理。

护士本身也应有合理的需要，并努力追求需要的满足，同时在工作中追求被患者需要的需要满足，以达到自我实现。

二、动机在临床护理中的应用

患者的求医动机、遵医嘱动机，与护士的护理工作密切相关，影响护理行为效果。护士必须记住，在患者、同事和自己的日常关系中，动机是起作用的。了解患者自身的动机将有助于护士在患者和医疗团队之间建立合作关系。护士应密切关注患者动机，识别患者可能存在的动机冲突，在护理工作中有意去引导患者转向切合实际的动机，积极配合医生、护士的治疗，尽快康复。

护士作为一个独立的个体，也有追求成就的动机、权力的动机、交往的动机等，同时也应意识到护理在患者康复过程中的意义，有机地把二者结合起来，以达到积极的护理效果。

练习题

1. 关于动机，下列表述错误的是（　　　）

　A. 动机不能被直接观察到　　　　　　　　B. 动机就是需要

　C. 可以通过个体对任务的选择等推断出动机　　D. 动机可以激发个体行为

2. 关于动机行为，下列表述正确的是（　　　）

　A. 动机引导的行为都有明确目标　　　　　B. 动机引导的行为都没有明确目标

　C. 不同的动机不会引发相同的行为　　　　D. 相同的动机引发的都是相同的行为

3. 饥饿会使个体做出觅食的活动，这是动机的（　　　）

　A. 导向功能　　　　B. 激活功能　　　　C. 调节和维持的功能　　　　D. 强化功能

4. 由于外部诱因引起的动机是（　　　）

　A. 外部动机　　　　B. 内部动机　　　　C. 交往动机　　　　D. 成就动机

5. 下列属于次要动机的是(　　)

　　A. 成就动机　　　　　　　B. 饥饿　　　　　　　　C. 性　　　　　　　　D. 爱好

6. 一般来说,由哪种动机支配的行为更具有持久性(　　)

　　A. 外部动机　　　　　　　B. 权力动机　　　　　　C. 内部动机　　　　　D. 交往动机

7. 根据马斯洛的需要层次理论,驱动力最强的是(　　)

　　A. 生理需要　　　　　　　B. 安全需要　　　　　　C. 归属需要　　　　　D. 自我实现需要

8. 关于需要,下列表述正确的是(　　)

　　A. 护士的个人需要对护理工作没有影响　　　　　B. 护士不需要考虑患者的个人需要

　　C. 护士应尽可能地满足患者的合理需要　　　　　D. 临床上不同患者的需要都一样

9. 关于动机,下列表述正确的是(　　)

　　A. 护士的个人动机对护理工作有影响　　　　　　B. 护士的成就动机很弱

　　C. 护士没有权力动机　　　　　　　　　　　　　D. 护士可以忽略个人动机

10. 马斯洛提出,人的最高级需要是(　　)

　　A. 生理需要　　　　　　　B. 安全需要　　　　　　C. 尊重需要　　　　　D. 自我实现需要

参考答案

第十三章 情　绪

━━━━━━ 学习目标 ━━━━━━

1. 掌握情绪的概念。
2. 熟悉情绪的发展。
3. 了解情绪的要素。

第一节　情绪的概念及要素

一、情绪的概念

情绪指对特定对象的强烈本能感觉的体验,通常伴随着身体的生理和行为变化。本能的意思是自动的,不需要有意识地思考的。情绪是以主观的愿望和需要为中介的一种心理活动,当客观事物或情景符合个体的愿望和需要时,就能引起积极的、肯定的情绪,反之,当客观事物或情景不符合个体的愿望和需要时,就会引起消极和否定的情绪。比如,长期卧病的患者经过康复训练,若可以自由活动就会感到高兴;若长期锻炼却效果不佳,难免会失望。有时客观事物或情景可能满足个体的某种需要,而不能满足另一种需要,甚至和其他需要相矛盾。因此,不少事物可能引起很复杂的情绪,比如百感交集、啼笑皆非、痛并快乐着等。

二、情绪的要素

情绪是一种混合的心理现象,由对刺激物的知觉、主观体验、生理唤醒、外部表现4种要素组成。

1. 对刺激物的知觉　首先要意识到刺激的存在,刺激才能对个体产生影响。刺激物可以是外部的自然或社会情境,也可以是内部的生理或心理感受。

2. 主观体验　是个体对不同情绪状态的自我感受。每一种情绪有不同的主观体验,它们代表了人的不同感受,如高兴和悲伤,构成了情绪的心理内容。情绪体验是一种复杂的主观感受,有时难以确定引起情绪体验的客观刺激是什么。而且,不同个体对同一刺激也可能产生不同的情绪,即使同一个体在不同时间、不同条件下对相同的刺激也会做出不同的情绪反应。比如个体在高兴时看夕阳可能"最美不过夕阳",在难过时就可能是"夕阳无限好,只是近黄昏。"

3. 生理唤醒　指的是情绪产生的生理反应,它涉及广泛的神经结构,如中枢神经系统的脑干、中央灰质、下丘脑等。不同情绪对生理的唤醒水平是不同的,如高兴愉快时心跳节律正常,暴怒时心跳加速、血压升高、呼吸频率增加,甚至出现间歇或停顿,痛苦时血管容积缩小,恐惧时胃的活动会暂停,消化液也停止分泌,汗腺分泌发生变化等。人在情绪状态下能自我知觉,但是不能很好地控制自己的情绪,因为主控情绪的自主神经系统一般不受个人意志控制。

4.外部表现 它是在情绪状态发生时身体各部分的动作量化形式,包括面部表情、姿态表情和言语表情。面部表情是所有面部肌肉变化组成的模式。如高兴时额眉平展、面颊上提、嘴角上翘。面部表情有泛文化性,同一种面部表情会被不同文化背景下的人们共同承认和使用,以表达相同的情绪体验。面部表情的识别研究还发现,最容易辨认的表情是快乐和痛苦,较难辨认的是恐惧和悲哀,最难辨认的是怀疑和怜悯。一般来说,情绪成分越复杂,表情越难辨认。姿态表情是指面部以外的身体其他部分的表情动作。例如高兴时手舞足蹈,悲痛时捶胸顿足,成功时趾高气扬,失败时垂头丧气等。姿态表情不具有跨文化性,并受不同文化的影响。言语表情是指情绪在言语的音调、节奏和速度等方面的表现。如激动时声音高尖,高兴时语调激扬、语速快,痛苦时语调低沉、节奏缓慢,紧张时语无伦次、音调有突然变化、常有言语中断和口误等。

第二节　情绪的发展及影响因素

一、情绪的发展

当一个孩子成长并发展他的运动技能时,他也发展了他的情绪,他的情绪不断分化和多样化。孩子2岁前的情绪变化发展较快。4~6周时,孩子在面对微笑时会有社交性微笑。3~4个月时,当你愤怒时,他会难过,听到大的噪声时他会好奇。5~7个月时,对陌生人会害怕,会被强噪声吓到。6~8个月时,会出现害羞情绪,有羞耻感,会厌恶一些事情。24个月时,各种情绪会更强烈,并学会调控自己的情绪。

二、影响情绪发展的因素

虽然弥漫性情绪可能在婴儿出生后不久就出现,但情绪的发展是成熟和学习的结果。影响情绪发展的因素主要有遗传、神经(脑)、认知-心理过程、应对方式和文化因素、环境条件、日常生活经验以及个人健康状况等。这些因素的相互作用使我们独一无二。

影响情绪发展的遗传因素之一是气质。气质广义上指的是生物行为上的个体差异,是表现在心理活动的强度、速度、灵活性与指向性等方面的一种稳定的心理特征,即我们平时所说的脾气、秉性。人的气质差异是先天形成的,受神经系统活动过程的特性制约,永远不会改变,它只是随着时间而发展。如孩子刚一出生时,有的孩子爱哭好动,有的孩子平稳安静,这种最先表现出来的差异就是气质差异。婴儿的这种气质差异也会影响他们与父母的关系,父母给予文静内敛的孩子比给予活泼爱动的孩子更多的鼓励。

气质是人的天性,无好坏之分。它只给人的言行涂上某种色彩,但不能决定人的社会价值,也不直接具有社会道德评价的含义。一个人的活泼与稳重不能决定他为人处事的方式。任何一种气质类型的人,既可以成为品德高尚、有益于社会的人,也可以成为品德败坏、有害于社会的人。气质影响人的择业,但不能决定一个人的成就,任何气质的人,只要经过自己的努力,都能在不同实践领域中取得成就,但也可能成为平庸无为的人。

现代的气质学说将气质分为4种典型的类型:胆汁质、多血质、黏液质、抑郁质。胆汁质这种类型的人感受性低、耐受性较高,情绪体验强烈、爆发迅猛、平息快速,思维灵活但粗枝大叶,精力旺盛、争强好斗、勇敢果断、为人热情直率、行动敏捷,但他们遇事常欠思量,鲁莽冒失、以感情用事,刚愎自用。多血质这种类型的人情感丰富、外露、但不稳定,思维敏捷、但不求甚解,活泼好动,善于交往,适应力强,但这种类型的人缺乏耐心和毅力,稳定性差,见异思迁。黏液质类型的人情绪平稳、表情平淡,思考问题周到细致,安静沉稳,自制力强,但这种类型的人缺乏生气,思维灵活性略差,行动迟缓,主动性差。抑郁质类型的人情绪体验深刻、细腻持久,情绪抑郁、多愁善感,思维敏锐,想象力丰富,自制力强,但这种类型的人举止缓慢、软弱胆小、优柔寡断。在现实生活中,单一气质的人并不多,大多数的人是4种气质的混合。

人与人之间存在个体差异,有些人快乐、开朗,吃饭、睡觉规律,适应新环境很快;另一些人可能慢热、孤僻、情绪化,需要更长的时间来适应新环境。有些婴儿爱挑剔、害怕,反应更强烈,这就需要护士在临床工作中能及时了解患儿的反应,了解孩子与父母或其他照顾者之间的依恋关系,有针对性地对待不同的患儿,更好地护理他们。

练习题

1. 由某种刺激引发的个体的主观心理感受称为( )
   A. 情绪　　　　　　B. 情操　　　　　　C. 品德　　　　　　D. 表情

2. 情绪是一种混合的心理现象,由哪4种要素组成( )
   A. 对刺激物的知觉、主观体验、生理唤醒、内部表现
   B. 对刺激物的知觉、主观体验、生理唤醒、外部表现
   C. 主观体验、生理唤醒、内部表现、外部表现
   D. 主观体验、肢体语言、内部表现、外部表现

3. 关于情绪,下列表述正确的是( )
   A. 相同的刺激,引发相同的情绪　　　　　　B. 相同的刺激,可引发不同的情绪
   C. 刺激满足个体需要,引发消极情绪　　　　D. 刺激不满足个体需要,引发积极情绪

4. 人在愤怒时心跳加速、血压升高、呼吸频率增加,这是情绪的( )
   A. 主观体验　　　　B. 外部表现　　　　C. 肢体语言　　　　D. 生理唤醒

5. 一般来说,表达情绪的主要方式是( )
   A. 眼部表情　　　　B. 言语表情　　　　C. 面部表情　　　　D. 嘴部表情

6. 关于情绪的外部表现,下列表述正确的是( )
   A. 面部表情具有泛文化性　　　　　　B. 姿态表情具有泛文化性
   C. 面部表情不具有泛文化性　　　　　D. 姿态表情不受文化习俗的影响

7. 影响孩子情绪发展的主要因素有( )
   A. 遗传　　　　　　B. 神经(脑)　　　　C. 认知-心理过程　　D. 以上都对

8. 婴儿的气质差异,是否会影响他与父母的关系( )
   A. 会　　　　　　　B. 不会　　　　　　C. 有时会　　　　　D. 有时不会

9. 下列不属于表情的是( )
   A. 面部表情　　　　B. 姿态表情　　　　C. 口干舌燥　　　　D. 言语表情

10. 婴儿在几周时会产生社交性表情( )
    A. 1~2周　　　　　B. 2~3周　　　　　C. 3~4周　　　　　D. 4~6周

参考答案

第十四章　记　忆

═══════ 学习目标 ═══════

1. 掌握记忆的概念。
2. 熟悉遗忘的进程。
3. 了解记忆的分类。

第一节　记忆的概念与分类

一、记忆的概念

记忆处理信息时,与电脑相似,即首先要写入文件,把文件存储到特定磁盘驱动器,需要时再从驱动器中提取出来。人感知过的事物、思考过的问题、体验过的情感或从事过的活动,都会在头脑中留下不同程度的印象,其中一些印象成为经验,能够保留相当长的时间,在一定条件下还能恢复,这就是记忆。

用信息加工的术语来讲,记忆就是人脑对外界输入的信息进行编码、存储和提取的过程。编码是对信息进行心理表征,以便将其保存在我们的记忆中(放入记忆中)。这是记忆的开初阶段,是获取个体经验的过程,相当于记忆中"记"的阶段。在记忆过程中,编码有不同的层次或水平,主要有视觉的、听觉的和语义的编码,不同的编码方式对记忆有不同的影响。

存储是将已编码的信息进行相对永久的存储,以便以后可以回忆(保存在内存中)的过程。存储是信息编码和提取的中间环节,在记忆过程中有着重要的作用。存储是一个积极的过程,存储的信息不是一成不变的,在内容和数量上都会发生变化。在数量方面,存储信息的数量随时间的推移而逐渐减少;在内容方面,存储的内容变得更加简略和概括,更加完整、合理和有意义,更加具体或者更加夸张和突出,不重要的细节将逐渐趋于消失。

提取是从短期或长期存储器中获取或回忆信息的过程(从记忆中恢复),是记忆过程的最后一个阶段,相当于记忆中"忆"的阶段。提取包括回忆和再认两种基本形式。经历过的事物不在眼前,能把它重新回想起来的过程,称为回忆。经历过的事物再度出现时,能把它认出来的过程,称为再认。例如考试时,填空题就是回忆的过程,选择题就是再认的过程。

记忆的 3 个基本过程是密切联系在一起的。一般来说,如果编码比较完善,存储得较好,提取就比较容易。

二、记忆的分类

根据信息保持时间的长短,将记忆分为感觉记忆、短时记忆和长时记忆。

1. 感觉记忆 当客观刺激停止作用后,感觉信息在一个极短的时间内被保存下来,这种记忆叫感觉记忆或感觉登记。感觉记忆就是个体从环境中接收信息的过程,是记忆系统的开始阶段,信息在大脑中的存储时间很短,为 0.25~4.00 s。感觉记忆有较大的容量,但只有能够引起个体注意并被及时识别的信息,才有机会进入短时记忆,那些没有被注意到的信息,很快就消失了。虽然信息在感觉记忆中保存的时间很短,但却很有用。在看电影和电视时,由于有感觉记忆,眼动和眨眼的时间并不影响我们知觉的连贯性。

2. 短时记忆 指的是能够短暂地保存有限的信息的记忆,是保持时间为 5 s~1 min 的记忆。它是感觉记忆和长时记忆的中间阶段,容量有限,为 7±2 个组块。影响短时记忆编码效果的因素有很多,觉醒状态即大脑皮质的兴奋水平,它直接影响记忆编码的效果。有研究表明,记忆广度的高峰在上午 10 点 30 分左右,整个下午都在下降,晚上效率最低。加工深度也是影响短时记忆编码的因素。最后,对记忆内容组块化或扩大每一个组块包含的信息量可以提高记忆的编码。例如:查一个电话号码,然后在忘记之前迅速拨号,如果你一遍又一遍地重复记忆,你就能在短期记忆中保持更长的时间,如果你更多地参与其中,比如在听讲座的同时也做笔记和复习,信息就会被编码到长时记忆中。

3. 长时记忆 是指保持时间超过 1 min,甚至终身的一种记忆。容量没有限制,信息的来源大部分是对短时记忆内容的加工,也有由于印象深刻而一次获得的。长时记忆中存储着我们过去的所有经验和知识,联结着人的心理活动的过去和现在,是我们学习、工作和生活的基本功能。编码时的意识状态影响长时记忆的编码。研究发现,有意编码的效果优于自动编码的效果。加工深度也影响长时记忆的编码。长时记忆中信息的提取取决于信息的存储方式和相关信息的干扰量。在信息储存中,准确度会发生变化,有时会失真。

感觉记忆、短时记忆和长时记忆不是非此即彼的记忆种类。它们的区别不仅仅是信息保持时间的长短或信息保存量的多少,而是在于它们在记忆系统的信息加工过程中处于不同的阶段,它们之间是持续的相互作用的过程。如图 14-1 所示,信息作用于感官,产生感觉记忆,感觉记忆中印象深刻的或经过加工的信息进入短时记忆中,其他信息消失;进入短时记忆中的信息,经过复述加工,成为长时记忆,未经过加工的信息消失,长时记忆中的信息也可提取到短时记忆中。

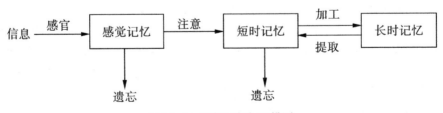

图 14-1 记忆三级加工模型

第二节 遗 忘

遗忘是指无法提取、回忆或识别已存储或仍存储在长期记忆中的信息。

一、遗忘的进程

最早研究遗忘的是德国心理学家艾宾浩斯。他以无意义音节为识记材料,让被试者重复学习,采用节省法测量记忆保持量,并将实验结果绘制成曲线,这就是著名的艾宾浩斯遗忘曲线(图14-2)。从图中可以看出,遗忘在学习之后立即开始,遗忘的过程最初进展得很快,以后逐渐缓慢。

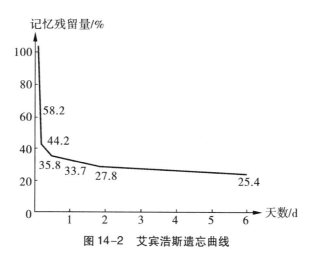

图14-2 艾宾浩斯遗忘曲线

二、遗忘的原因

干扰学说认为,遗忘是由于其他相关记忆而导致记忆受阻,无法回忆起特定信息。比如同一天要参加几场考试,为考试准备的内容很可能会混淆和遗忘。前摄抑制和倒摄抑制可以很好地证明干扰说。

前摄抑制是先学习的材料对识记和回忆后学习的材料的干扰作用。倒摄抑制是后学习的材料对识记和回忆先学习材料的干扰作用。比如背诵一首诗歌,诗歌的前半部分和后半部分一般识记得快,记得牢,中间部分识记得慢,忘得快,就是因为中间部分受前摄抑制和倒摄抑制的双重影响。这也提醒我们学习时要注意材料的序列位置,打乱学习材料的顺序进行学习,中间部分也要多加复习巩固,以防遗忘。

失忆症是大脑受到打击或损伤后暂时或永久的记忆丧失,这可能是由于疾病或创伤引起的。

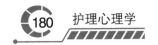

练习题

1. 信息保持在 1 min 以上甚至终身的记忆称为(　　)
   A. 短时记忆　　　　　　B. 感觉记忆　　　　　　C. 长时记忆　　　　　　D. 永远记忆

2. 短时记忆容量有限,为了使其包含更多的信息,可以采取的方式是(　　)
   A. 组块　　　　　　　　B. 复述　　　　　　　　C. 注意　　　　　　　　D. 感觉登记

3. 感觉记忆的信息,只有受到哪种刺激才会进入短时记忆,其他都被遗忘(　　)
   A. 感觉　　　　　　　　B. 注意　　　　　　　　C. 知觉　　　　　　　　D. 思维

4. 短时记忆的容量有几个组块(　　)
   A. 6±2　　　　　　　　B. 7±2　　　　　　　　C. 6±3　　　　　　　　D. 7±3

5. 考试时,对于选择题,学生主要的记忆活动是(　　)
   A. 回忆　　　　　　　　B. 识记　　　　　　　　C. 保持　　　　　　　　D. 再认

6. 关于长时记忆中信息的保持,下列表述错误的是(　　)
   A. 存储信息的数量随时间的推移而逐渐减少　　B. 存储的内容变得更加简略和概括
   C. 重要的细节将逐渐趋于消失　　　　　　　　D. 不重要的细节将逐渐趋于消失

7. 记忆有 3 个基本过程,它们是编码、存储和(　　)
   A. 遗忘　　　　　　　　B. 注意　　　　　　　　C. 联想　　　　　　　　D. 提取

8. 学习后立刻睡觉,保持的效果比学习后再继续其他活动保持的效果好,这在因为(　　)
   A. 无前摄抑制的影响　　B. 无倒摄抑制的影响　C. 过度学习　　　　　　D. 记忆恢复现象

9. 艾宾浩斯发现,遗忘的进程是(　　)
   A. 先快后慢　　　　　　B. 先慢后快　　　　　　C. 时快时慢　　　　　　D. 一样快

10. 根据艾宾浩斯的发现,复习时应(　　)
   A. 分散复习与集中复习相结合　　　　　　B. 有意复习和无意复习相结合
   C. 及时复习　　　　　　　　　　　　　　D. 合理分配复习时间

参考答案

第十五章　人　格

▨▨▨▨▨·学习目标·▨▨▨▨▨

1. 掌握人格发展的3种理论。
2. 熟悉影响人格的因素。
3. 了解人格的定义,研究人格的目的。

第一节　人格的定义及研究意义

一、人格的定义

人格是个体思维、感觉和行为的特征模式。人们通常认为,人格来自一个人的内心,并在整个生命中保持相当一致。

什么是人格? 17世纪的哲学家托马斯·霍布斯认为,人类天生就是自私的。他认为,在自然状态下的生活是"肮脏、野蛮和短暂的"。18世纪的政治哲学家让·雅克·卢梭不同意这种观点,他坚持认为人天生就是善良的,理性的人自由行动会促进所有人的福祉。

这两种观点之间的争论在人格理论中仍然存在。西格蒙德·弗洛伊德认为,人类生来就有冲动,如果文明要生存,就必须加以控制。卡尔·罗杰斯认为,人们在摆脱了不必要的束缚后,才会寻求美好而崇高的目标。

哪种观点是正确的? 从内心深处来说,我们是好、坏,两者兼而有之,还是两者都不是? 人类人格的基本性质是什么?

人格一词来自拉丁语"persona",意思是"面具"。在古希腊和古罗马的戏剧中,演员戴着面具来表明他们的角色。然而,与面具不同的是,人格一词意味着某种稳定的东西。人格包括一个人的行为与其他人的行为不同的所有方式,尤其是在社交场合(学习、记忆、感觉或运动技能的差异通常不被视为人格)。

二、研究人格的意义

(1)为更好地了解患者疾病提供重要指导。

(2)更好地照顾每位患者。

(3)深入了解个别护士如何处理他或她在照顾患者方面的角色。

第二节　人格的发展

人类可以根据他们的行为、感觉或以特定方式思考的可能性来描述,称为特质。特质是人格的基本单位。

一、行为主义者认为人格特质的3个方面

1. 外向性与内向性　外向的人善于交际,渴望刺激和变化,因此很容易感到无聊。他们更有可能冒险并寻求刺激。艾森克认为,这是因为他们继承了一个兴奋不足的神经系统,因此寻求刺激以达到最佳刺激水平。相反,内向的人则处于这个量表的另一端,安静而内向。他们已经过度兴奋并关闭了感觉和刺激。内向的人,习惯计划他们的行动并控制他们的情绪。他们往往是严肃的、可靠的和悲观的。

2. 神经质　一个人的神经质程度取决于交感神经系统的反应。一个稳定的人的神经系统通常对压力情况的反应较小,能保持冷静和头脑清醒。相反,神经质高的人会更加不稳定,容易对刺激反应过度,可能会很容易担心、愤怒或恐惧。他们过于情绪化,一旦心烦意乱就很难平静下来。

3. 精神质　埃森克后来增加了第三个特质/维度——精神质。例如,缺乏同理心、残忍、孤独、好斗和容易引起麻烦。这与高水平的睾酮有关。

根据艾森克的说法,神经质(稳定与不稳定)和外向性与内向性这两个维度结合起来形成了多种人格特征。

二、精神分析方法

人格发展取决于生命前5年本能(自然)和环境(父母影响)的相互作用。童年时期的环境和父母经历会影响一个人成年后的性格。例如,在生命的前2年,被忽视(喂养不足)或过度保护(过度喂养)的婴儿可能会变成一个口欲大的人。

(一)西格蒙德·弗洛伊德的性心理阶段

1. 第一阶段口欲期　在口腔阶段,从出生到大约1岁,婴儿从口腔刺激中获得强烈的快乐,特别是在吸吮母亲的乳房时。根据弗洛伊德的说法,在这个阶段沉迷的人继续从饮食和吸烟中获得极大的乐趣,并且还可能在依靠和独立方面令人有持久的担忧。

2. 第二阶段肛门期　大约在2岁时,儿童进入肛门阶段,此时他们从排便的感觉中获得性心理快感。如果如厕训练过于严格或过于宽松,孩子会在这个阶段变得固执。固执于肛门阶段的人会在生活中"拖后腿"——慢条斯理、小气、固执;或者也可能走向相反的极端,变得凌乱和浪费。

3. 第三阶段性器期　3岁开始,儿童进入性器期。弗洛伊德说:"儿童由3岁起,其性生活即类同于成人的性生活"。所不同的是:①因生殖器未成熟,以致没有稳固的组织性;②倒错现象的存在;③整个冲动较为薄弱。这里,弗洛伊德所说的3岁后的所谓"性生活"又指的什么呢? 主要是指出现男孩的恋母情结转换期,女孩也产生恋父情结。也就是说,到了这个阶段,儿童变得依恋于父母中异性的一方。

4. 第四阶段潜伏期　随着建立较强的抵御恋母情结或恋父情结的情感,儿童进入潜伏期。弗洛伊德认为,儿童进入潜伏期,其性的发展便呈现一种停滞的或退化的现象,可能完全缺乏,也可能不完全缺乏。这个时期,口欲期、肛门期的感觉,性器期的恋母(恋父)情结的各种记忆都逐渐被遗

忘,被压抑的性感差不多一扫而光,因此,潜伏期是一个相当平静的时期。

5.第五阶段生殖期 经过暂时的潜伏期,青春期的风暴就来到了,从年龄上讲,女孩约从11岁,男孩约从13岁开始进入生殖期。按照弗洛伊德及其女儿安娜·弗洛伊德的观点,首先,青春期的发展,个体的最重要的任务是要从父母那里摆脱自己。同时,到了生殖期,个体容易产生性的冲动,也容易产生同成人的抵触情绪和冲动(表15-1)。

表15-1 西格蒙德弗洛伊德的性心理阶段

阶段	年龄段	特征
口欲期	0~1岁	儿童从口腔相关的活动中获得愉悦感,例如用嘴吃和吸。他们喜欢把东西放到嘴里
肛门期	2~3岁	儿童开始进行如厕训练
性器期	3~6岁	男孩更依恋母亲,女孩更依恋父亲
潜伏期	6岁至青春期	儿童会花费更多的时间与同性别的同伴互动
生殖期	青春期之后	容易被异性同伴吸引

(二)人格的结构

根据弗洛伊德的说法,我们的人格是由两种力量之间的冲突发展而来的:我们的生物攻击性和寻求快乐的驱动力与我们对这些驱动力的内部(社会化)控制。我们的性格是我们努力平衡这两种竞争力量的结果[弗洛伊德建议我们可以通过在我们的脑海中想象3个相互作用的系统来理解这一点。他称之为本我、自我和超我。根据弗洛伊德的说法,我们的性格是由两种力量之间的冲突发展而来的:本我和超我。我们的性格(自我)是我们努力平衡这两种竞争力量的结果]。

(三)防御机制

1.压抑 是有动机地将某些东西转移到无意识中拒绝不可接受的想法、欲望和记忆。例如,有不可接受的性冲动的人可能没有意识到这一点。弗洛伊德坚持认为,人们会压抑痛苦、创伤性的记忆。被压抑的情景被从意识中移除,但不会被遗忘。弗洛伊德曾经把一个被压抑的情景比作一个吵闹的人被赶出一个房间,但是他继续敲门,试图重新进去。

2.否认 拒绝相信不愉快的信息("这不可能发生")是否认。压抑是从意识中清除信息的动机,而否认则是断言信息不正确,通常伴随着实现愿望的幻想。例如,有酗酒问题的人可能会坚持说:"我不是酒鬼。我可以喝酒,也可以不喝酒。"即将离婚的人可能会坚持认为婚姻一切顺利。即将被解雇的人可能会认为他们在工作中非常成功。

3.合理化 当人们试图证明他们的行为是合理的时,他们会使用合理化。例如,一个想去看电影的学生说:"无论如何,更多的学习对我没有任何好处。"不公平地占他人便宜的人会说:"学会处理失望会让他成为一个更好的人。"

4.替代 通过将行为或思想从其自然目标转向威胁较小的目标,替代让人们以较少的焦虑参与行为。例如,如果你对你的雇主或教授生气,你可能会对其他人大吼大叫。

5.投射 将自己不受欢迎的特征归因于他人被称为投射。如果有人告诉你不要生气,你可能会回答:"我不生气!生气的就是你!"暗示其他人有你的缺点可能会使这些缺点看起来不那么具有威胁性。例如,偷偷喜欢色情的人可能会指责其他人喜欢色情。然而,研究发现,使用投射的人通常不会减少他们的焦虑或对自己错误的认识。

6.反向形成 为了避免意识到某些弱点,人们有时会使用反向形成来表现自己与真实情况的

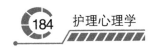

对立面。换句话说,他们走向了相反的极端。一个因怀疑自己的宗教信仰而烦恼的人可能会试图让其他人皈依该信仰;具有极度攻击倾向的人可能会加入一个致力于防止暴力的团体。

7.升华　将性或攻击性的能量转化为文化上可接受的甚至令人钦佩的行为。根据弗洛伊德的说法,升华让某人在不承认其存在的情况下表达一种冲动。例如,绘画和雕塑可能代表了性冲动的升华。有人可能会通过成为外科医生来升华攻击性冲动。升华是一种假设的与社会建设性行为相关的防御机制。但是,如果画家的真正动机是性,而外科医生的真正动机是暴力,那么这些动机确实被隐藏得很好。

三、人本主义的理论

人本主义的理论关注个人对世界的个人看法、自我概念和发挥最大潜能的能力。人们对自己的生活和行为负责,有改变态度和行为的自由和意愿。

人本主义理论的哲学根源在于现象学和存在主义,有些人会说它们比"心理学"更"哲学"。他们关注的是特别的和独一无二的人类特征,特别是经验、独特性、意义、自由和选择。作为人,我们有自己的第一手经验,特别是罗杰斯的理论是围绕自我概念的。

罗杰斯和马斯洛的共同点是他们对人性的积极评价,相信个人的成长潜力(自我实现)。但是,虽然马斯洛的理论通常被称为"存在的心理学"(自我实现本身就是目的,并且处于需求层次的顶峰),但罗杰斯的理论是"成为的心理学"(它侧重于成为"功能齐全的人"的过程)。

根据托伦斯和乔丹的理论,马斯洛对人类需求的描述强调了生物科学在护理理论和实践中的核心作用。护士每天都会遇到健康状况不佳和疾病的个体,因此临床护理实践是围绕个体对这些健康问题的生理和心理反应而形成的。尽管护理实践显然具有超越治疗疾病的作用(例如健康教育和促进),但其主要关注点仍然是生病的人。托伦斯和乔丹认为,从更广泛的角度来看,护理旨在帮助解决缺陷和成长需求,但它必须确保满足直接的生理和安全需求。如果护士与患者的关系在满足这些基本需求方面是有效的,那么它就可以在满足更高层次的需求方面提供帮助。然而,人们之所以成为患者,往往是因为疾病干扰了他们利用自己的资源满足较低层次需求的能力。

自我概念和与自我相关的体验是人格发展的核心。人们的运动方向基本上是朝着自我实现的方向发展。罗杰斯进一步将自我分为两类:理想自我和真实自我。卡尔·罗杰斯的以人为本理论认为理想自我与真实自我如果不一致,可能导致混乱、紧张和适应不良的行为。

练习题

1.提出人类天生就是自私的心理学家是(　　　)
　A.托马斯　　　　　　　B.班杜拉　　　　　　　C.罗杰斯　　　　　　　D.米勒

2.艾森克研究发现,哪项特质与睾酮的分泌有关(　　　)
　A.内外向性　　　　　　B.神经质　　　　　　　C.宜人性　　　　　　　D.精神质

3.个体的思想、情感及行为的特有整合,其中包含区别于他人的稳定而统一的心理品质是(　　　)
　A.性格　　　　　　　　B.气质　　　　　　　　C.能力　　　　　　　　D.人格

4.提出人类天生就是善良的心理学家是(　　　)
　A.托马斯　　　　　　　B.班杜拉　　　　　　　C.卢梭　　　　　　　　D.米勒

5.个体潜意识地阻止有关自己痛苦的事实进入意识,这种自我防御机制是(　　　)
　A.压抑　　　　　　　　B.否认　　　　　　　　C.自居作用　　　　　　D.投射作用

6.具有极度攻击倾向的人可能会加入一个致力于防止暴力的团体,这种自我防御机制是(　　)

  A.压抑　　　　　　　　B.否认　　　　　　　　C.反向形成　　　　　　D.投射作用

7.健康的人是自我实现的人,而人的基本需要的满足是在人际关系中实现的,这种观点的提出者是(　　)

  A.罗杰斯　　　　　　　B.马斯洛　　　　　　　C.奥尔波特　　　　　　D.班杜拉

8.根据弗洛伊德的说法,年龄在3~6岁之间的学龄前儿童会发展出性兴趣,并且对衣服和发型产生兴趣,这属于性心理阶段的(　　)

  A.肛门期　　　　　　　B.性器期　　　　　　　C.生殖期　　　　　　　D.潜伏期

9.儿童在排便过程中获得心理快感,这属于性心理阶段中的(　　)

  A.肛门期　　　　　　　B.性器期　　　　　　　C.生殖期　　　　　　　D.潜伏期

10.关注个人对世界的个人看法、自我概念和发挥最大潜能的能力,这是以下哪种人格理论(　　)

  A.人本主义理论　　　　B.生理学理论　　　　　C.行为主义理论　　　　D.心理动力学理论

参考答案

第十六章　疾　病

▨▨▨▨▨ 学习目标 ▨▨▨▨▨

1. 掌握影响疾病的因素、恶性肿瘤患者的心理反应。
2. 熟悉疾病的分类、患者角色适应困难的表现、护士承担的角色。
3. 了解疾病的基本概念、患者角色特点。

第一节　概　述

一、基本概念

健康是指机体在生命活动过程中,通过神经-体液调节,各器官的功能、代谢和形态结构维持着正常的协调关系,而机体与变化着的外界环境保持相对平衡。

1946 年世界卫生组织成立时,在宪章中明确提出:"健康不仅仅是没有疾病和身体的虚弱现象,而是一种身体上、心理上和社会上的完美状态。"1990 年世界卫生组织对健康做出新的定义,即"健康不仅仅是没有疾病,而且包括躯体健康、心理健康、社会适应良好和道德健康。"

病感是指个体能够感到有病或不适的主观体验,常常无法直接验证,影响其身心状态,感觉不舒服或有某种痛苦,伴有不同程度的生理、心理、社会功能的失调,并由此产生求医行为。病感可能是由于某种疾病所引起的疼痛等躯体反应,也可以是受心理、社会等因素影响,导致个体出现生理反应和心理反应。

疾病是指个体由于致病因素的侵袭,正常的生理、心理活动偏离常态,机体系统的功能协调有序性被破坏,社会适应性受损。在多数疾病中,机体对病因所引起的损害发生一系列抗损害反应,结果可能是疾病痊愈或残疾,甚至个体死亡。自稳调节的紊乱、损害和抗损害反应,表现为疾病过程中各种复杂的功能、代谢和形态结构的异常变化,而这些变化又可使机体各器官系统之间以及机体与外界环境之间的协调关系发生障碍,从而引起各种症状、体征和行为异常,特别是对环境适应能力和劳动能力的减弱甚至丧失。

疾病与病感既有区别又有联系。疾病是指人体的器官组织或心理受到损害,出现病症、相应的体征或行为特征,实验室检查有阳性发现,患者的社会功能下降。病感是一种主观体验。个体有了病感可能会出现求医行为,但病感不一定是疾病。但有些疾病尽管已经很严重,但是患者并没有病感,如常规体检发现的癌症。

患者又称病人,有狭义和广义之分。狭义的患者是指患有各种躯体疾病、心身疾病或精神障碍等的人,不论求医与否,均称为患者,也包括那些只有病感,在临床上未发现躯体病理改变的人。广义的患者是指接受医疗卫生服务的所有对象,包括健康的人。

二、疾病的分类

按照疾病发病的急缓和进展的快慢,可将疾病分为急性病和慢性病。

急性病指发病急剧、病情发展很快、症状较重的疾病,如急性阑尾炎等。按照其病情可分为轻度、中度和重度。轻度往往指局部小的损伤或病变,对身体的影响不大;中度往往是指已经影响身体的功能或行为的病变;重度则是指严重影响身体的功能或行为的病变。对于轻度的患者,可以在家自行进行短暂的处理,比如不严重的咳嗽、少量的腹泻、较轻的皮肤擦伤等;如果经过处理好转就不需要去医院,如果处理后不见好转或加重了,则应该去医院诊治。对于中度和重度的病情就要尽早或紧急去医院就诊。

慢性病是一种渐变性的、症状不很强烈的疾病,起病隐匿,病程长且病情迁延不愈,持续时间较长,6 个月或更长时间,病因复杂,影响患者劳动能力和生活质量,如糖尿病、心脏病等。

三、影响疾病的因素

1. 年龄 疾病的发生跟年龄有一定的关系。随着年龄的增长,人患病的可能性就越大。多项研究发现,65 岁以后阿尔茨海默病的发病率会逐渐增加,七八十岁是比较集中的发病阶段。

2. 性别 在某些疾病上,性别不同,发病率则不同。研究表明女性抑郁症的发病率是男性的 2 倍。同时不同性别易患癌症的种类不同,如女性的子宫癌、男性的前列腺癌。

3. 经济状况 个体的经济状况在一定程度上影响其物质生活水平,经济较差,可导致摄入的蛋白质、脂肪、维生素等较少,导致营养不良。经济较好,可摄入过量的食物,导致体重超重,从而影响健康。

4. 社会文化 社会文化是与基层广大群众生产和生活实际紧密相连,由基层群众创造,具有地域、民族或群体特征,并对社会群体施加广泛影响的各种文化现象和文化活动的总称。不同国家、不同民族有不同的社会文化,不同社会文化对同一疾病的看法不同,不同时代对同一疾病的看法也不尽相同。

5. 人格 人格完善是健康的重要标志,人格完善是指有健全统一的人格,能力、性格、气质、兴趣、世界观等方面能和谐平衡发展,不存在明显缺陷和偏差。研究发现,A 型行为类型的人易患冠心病,C 型行为类型的人容易患上恶性肿瘤。

6. 生活方式 据统计,吸烟、酗酒、药物滥用、过量饮食和肥胖、运动不足等不良的生活方式已经成为影响人类健康的重要因素。

7. 遗传 遗传性因素直接致病主要是通过遗传物质基因的突变和染色体畸变。基因突变引起分子病,如血友病;染色体畸变引起染色体病,目前已达到数百种,如性染色体畸变导致的两性畸形等。

四、疾病阶段

美国学者 Suchman 通过观察医疗活动的程序,把疾病分为 5 个阶段:症状体验、承担患者角色、获取医疗服务、依赖性患病角色、痊愈和康复。

1. 症状体验 在这个阶段,个体感觉身体有不适感,由于缺乏医学知识,往往自己不能诊断出问题。这个时候,患者往往会产生 3 个方面的症状,分别是症状的身体体验、认知方面和情绪上的反应。在这一阶段末期,往往能够意识到这是某种疾病的症状。

2. **承担患者角色** 如果症状持续存在,那么个体将承担患病的角色,并寻求家人或其他人的支持。然后他就会从正常的职责和角色期望中解脱出来,不在履行正常角色所承担的义务和责任。在这个阶段,患者会产生不良情绪,如恐惧、焦虑、愤怒等,患者会出现延迟就医行为。

3. **获取医疗服务** 在这个阶段,患者将主动或在他人教促后寻求治疗,医生利用专业知识判断是否患病。如果患者接受医生的诊断,患者将遵医嘱接受治疗。患者通常情况下,会问 3 种类型的信息,是否属于疾病、对症状的解释和预后情况。有的患者对医生的诊断持怀疑的态度,从而拒绝接受治疗。

4. **依赖性患病角色** 患者都渴望尽快恢复健康,所以都能积极接受治疗和护理。患者渴望得到周围人的帮助和关心,对医生和护士产生依赖心理和行为。甚至有些患者对疾病过于关心,过度依赖医院环境,在治疗好转或痊愈后,不愿意从患者角色转为常态角色,不愿意离开医务工作者。

5. **痊愈和康复** 在这个阶段,疾病症状消失,患者开始恢复健康状态,一般情况下,患者能重新回到以往的生活状态中,但有些疾病,可导致患者社会功能长期下降。

五、疾病对患者、家庭和社会的影响

疾病不是一个孤立的生活事件,会引起患者及其家庭发生一些变化。这些变化因为疾病的类型、严重程度和持续时间、治疗费用,以及患者生活方式的改变、角色的改变和调整等有所不同。

(一)疾病对患者的影响

1. **个人行为与情绪方面的影响** 一般来说,疾病造成的个体行为与情绪改变可因疾病的性质、患者及他人对该病的态度的不同而有所不同。通常,短期的、无生命危险的疾病不会引起患者太大的情绪和行为变化,但是重病,尤其是威胁生命的疾病则可引起强烈的行为和情绪变化,如焦虑、震惊、愤怒等。

2. **个人自主性与生活方式的影响** 疾病通常可降低个人的自主性,而出现更多的依从或遵医行为。

3. **对身体形象产生的影响** 一些疾病可引起患者身体形象的改变,从而导致患者和家属产生一系列心理反应。反应的程度取决于外表改变的类型、患者与家属的适应能力、外表改变的突然性和支持系统是否健全。

4. **对自我概念的影响** 自我概念受很多因素的影响,如身体某部分或功能的缺失、疼痛、依赖他人、参与社会活动能力缺乏等。

(二)疾病对家庭的影响

1. **经济影响** 个体患病后,需要到医院就诊或住院治疗,甚至是手术治疗,这些都会增加家庭开支,给家庭带来一定的经济负担。有的患者为了减轻家庭的经济负担,会选择放弃治疗,甚至产生极端的行为,从而影响疾病的治疗和康复。如果患者是家庭经济收入的主要来源者,会加重家庭的经济负担,对家庭产生更为严重的影响。

2. **家庭成员心理压力过大** 患者家属不仅要承担患者原有的家庭角色,而且还要投入大量的时间和精力来照顾患者,使家庭成员的负担加重,并产生相应的心理压力。

3. **家庭角色的改变** 疾病对家庭角色变化的影响可能是短期的或长期的,这取决于疾病的性质。短期疾病对患者和家庭的功能影响较小。

(三)疾病对社会的影响

1. **降低社会生产力** 每个人在工作时都以其社会角色对社会做出贡献,当个体转变患者角色后,暂时或长期免除了社会责任,不能承担原有社会角色时,必定降低社会生产力。

2. 消耗社会医疗资源　诊断和治疗疾病都会消耗一定的社会医疗资源。

3. 造成传染，威胁他人健康　某些传染性疾病，如肝炎、结核等，如不采取适当的措施，会在人群中传播，感染他人，影响他人健康。

第二节　患者角色与护士承担的角色

一、患者角色

当一个人被确诊患有某种疾病时，他就获得了另外一个角色，即患者角色，也称患者身份。

(一)患者角色的特点

1. 社会角色退化　个体患病后，可以从原来的社会角色中解脱出来，他原本承担的社会与家庭责任、权利和义务被酌情免除，并可根据疾病性质及严重程度，获得休息或接受医疗帮助。

2. 自控能力下降　个体患病后会出现软弱依赖，情绪多变，意志力减退和自我调节能力、适应能力、控制能力下降等，渴望得到照顾。

3. 求助愿望强烈　处于疾病状态中的个体，都希望摆脱疾病的痛苦，力求痊愈。为了减少病痛的折磨和尽快恢复健康，患者会积极寻求他人的帮助。

4. 合作意愿增强　患者都渴望尽快康复，所以都会积极地接受诊断、治疗和护理，与医务工作者、亲友或其他患者主动、密切合作，争取早日痊愈。

5. 康复后有承担病前社会责任的义务　患者在康复后，都要走出患者角色，恢复原有的各种社会角色，承担原来的社会责任。

(二)患者角色适应困难

个体患病后，一般情况下，患者都会慢慢适应患者角色，称为角色适应。但是，还有些患者在由以往的社会角色进入患者角色时发生困难，或在康复时由患者角色转变为健康人角色发生困难，这些表现都称为患者角色适应困难。常见的类型如下。

1. 患者角色冲突　患者角色冲突是指患者在角色转换时不能够或不愿意放弃原有的社会角色行为，因而与其病前的各种角色发生心理冲突而引起行为的不协调。患者常表现为焦虑不安、愤怒、烦恼、茫然和悲伤。这种情况多见于社会或家庭责任较多，而且事业心、责任心比较强的人。

2. 患者角色强化　有的患者在进入患者角色以后，表现出对疾病状态的过分认同，甚至对疾病康复后要承担的社会角色感到恐惧不安，称为患者角色强化。这些患者主要表现为对自身所患疾病的过分关心，过度依赖医院环境；在治疗好转或痊愈后，不愿从患者角色转为常态角色，往往不承认病情好转或痊愈，不愿出院，不愿离开医务工作者，不愿重返原来的工作、学习和生活环境。

3. 患者角色缺如　患者角色缺如是指患者意识不到或者对疾病持否定态度，对自己疾病的严重程度过于忽视，拒绝按患者角色行事。有的人可能因为对突然患病缺乏心理准备，不相信自己会患病，满不在乎；还有的人对疾病的严重程度和后果过于忽视，或者因为经济紧张害怕花钱等，其后果可能是拒绝就医，贻误了治疗，使病情进一步恶化。

4. 患者角色减退　患者角色减退是指患者进入患者角色后，疾病还未痊愈，由于某种原因导致患者过早地退出患者角色回到社会常态角色，与角色强化的情形相反。常常是因为家庭、工作中的突发事件，比如亲人突然生病、工作单位考评考核、晋升职称等。角色减退多发生疾病中期，也是一种患者角色冲突的表现，对疾病的进一步治疗和康复不利。

5. 患者角色恐惧 患者角色恐惧是指患者对疾病缺乏正确的认识和态度,患病后表现为对疾病的过度担忧、恐惧等消极的情绪,对疾病的后果夸大其词,对进一步治疗缺乏信心,对康复过度悲观、失望。患者往往四处求医,希望马上从疾病中解脱,因而病急乱投医,甚至滥用药物。

6. 患者角色隐瞒 患者角色隐瞒是指由于某种原因患者不能或不愿承担疾病所造成的影响及后果,故而隐瞒疾病真相。如艾滋病患者、心理障碍者对自己角色的保密,还有患者为宽慰家人,避免家人为之担忧而隐瞒自己的疾病。

7. 患者角色假冒 患者角色假冒是指并无疾病,但为了逃脱某种社会责任和义务或为获得某些利益而诈病,假冒患者角色。

二、恶性肿瘤患者的心理反应

1. 休克-恐惧期 当患者初次得知自己恶性肿瘤时会产生一个震惊时期,称为"诊断休克"。患者反应强烈,极力否认恶性肿瘤的诊断,表现为震惊和恐惧,同时会出现一些躯体反应如心悸、眩晕及昏厥,甚至木僵状态。此期短暂,历时数日或数周。

2. 否认-怀疑期 患者从剧烈的情绪反应中平静下来后,常借助于否认机制来保护自己,患者开始怀疑医师的诊断是否正确,到处求医,希望能找到一位能否定恶性肿瘤诊断的医师,希望有奇迹发生;或千方百计探索民间治疗的秘方,采用一些不切实际的治疗方案,以求生存。

3. 愤怒-沮丧期 当患者渐渐接受恶性肿瘤的诊断时,便会陷入极度的痛苦之中,情绪变得异常脆弱,易激惹、愤怒,有时还会伴有攻击行为;患者常常感到悲哀、沮丧甚至绝望,有的患者甚至会产生轻生的念头或自杀的行为。

4. 接受-适应期 患病的事实无法改变,患者能冷静地面对事实,心境平静,治疗合作。但多数患者很难恢复到患病前的心境,常常轻度抑郁、焦虑;晚期时,患者常处于无望及无助状态,常常消极被动应付。

三、护士承担的角色

1. 照顾者 在临床工作中,照顾患者,为患者提供直接的护理服务,满足患者生理、心理和社会各方面的需要,是护士的首要职责。

2. 管理者 每个护士都有管理的职责。护理领导者管理人力资源和物资资源,组织护理工作的实施,管理的目的是提高护理的质量和效率;普通护士管理患者和病区环境,促进患者早日康复。

3. 教育者 护士在许多场合行使教育者的职能。在医院,对患者和家属进行卫生宣教,讲解有关疾病的治疗、护理和预防知识,同时有带教护生的任务;在社区,向居民宣传预防疾病、保持健康的知识和方法;在护理学校,向护理学生传授专业知识和技能。

4. 患者权益的保护者 护士有责任帮助患者理解来自各种途径的健康信息,补充必要信息,帮助患者做出正确的选择;保护患者的权益不受侵犯和损害。

5. 协调者和合作者 护士与护理对象、家庭和其他健康专业人员需要紧密合作,相互配合和支持,更好地满足护理对象的需要。

6. 示范者 护士应在预防保健、促进健康生活方式等方面起示范作用,如不吸烟、讲究卫生、加强体育锻炼等。

7. 咨询者 护士有责任为护理对象提供健康信息,给予预防保健等专业指导。

8. 研究者 开展护理研究,解决复杂的临床问题,以及在护理教育、护理管理等领域中遇到的有关问题,完善护理理论,推动护理专业的发展。

9. 改革者和创业者 护士应适应社会发展的需要,不断改革护理的服务方式,扩大护理工作范围和职责,推动护理事业的发展。

练习题

1. 人在社会中扮演多种角色,其行为应随时间、环境不同进行调整,这是(　　　)
   A. 角色期待　　　　　　B. 角色转换　　　　　　C. 角色冲突　　　　　　D. 角色矛盾

2. 进入患者角色的根本原因是(　　)
   A. 从原有的社会角色中解脱　　　　　　　B. 环境发生了改变
   C. 患病　　　　　　　　　　　　　　　D. 处于被帮助的地位

3. 患者由于工作繁忙或者家庭责任而不能安心治疗,这是(　　)
   A. 患者角色冲突　　B. 患者角色缺如　　C. 患者角色消退　　D. 患者角色隐瞒

4. 某人已被确诊为癌症,而本人否认自己有病,这是(　　)
   A. 患者角色冲突　　　　　　　　　　　B. 患者角色缺如
   C. 患者角色消退　　　　　　　　　　　D. 患者角色隐瞒

5. 医生判断患者疾病已经康复,但患者本人认为自己还需要住院治疗,这是(　　)
   A. 患者角色冲突　　　　　　　　　　　B. 患者角色缺如
   C. 患者角色消退　　　　　　　　　　　D. 患者角色强化

6. 关于病感和疾病的说法,下列错误的是(　　)
   A. 两者有区别有联系　　　　　　　　　B. 病感是一种主观体验
   C. 病感不一定是疾病　　　　　　　　　D. 所有的疾病都有病感

7. 癌症患者听到癌症的诊断后,出现心理反应的顺序是(　　)
   A. 否认-怀疑期,愤怒-沮丧期,接受-适应期,休克-恐惧期
   B. 否认-怀疑期,休克-恐惧期,愤怒-沮丧期,接受-适应期
   C. 休克-恐惧期,愤怒-沮丧期,接受-适应期,否认-怀疑期
   D. 休克-恐惧期,否认-怀疑期,愤怒-沮丧期,接受-适应期

8. 护士承担的角色,不包括下列哪一项(　　)
   A. 管理者　　　　　　B. 照顾者　　　　　　C. 诊断者　　　　　　D. 研究者

9. 疾病对患者的影响,下列说法不正确的是(　　)
   A. 影响正常社会角色的扮演　　　　　　B. 影响自我概念
   C. 影响自主性和生活方式　　　　　　　D. 加重家庭经济负担

10. 影响疾病的因素,不包括下列哪一项(　　)
    A. 身高　　　　　　B. 经济状况　　　　　　C. 社会文化　　　　　　D. 年龄

参考答案

第十七章 残 疾

1. 掌握残疾的概念。
2. 熟悉残疾的分类。
3. 了解残疾的心理反应。

第一节 概 述

一、残疾的概念

残疾是指身体或精神的任何状况(损伤)使有这种状况的人更难进行某些活动(活动限制)以及与周围世界的互动(参与限制)。几乎每个人都可能在人生的某个时刻经历某种形式的残疾——暂时的或永久的。残疾人也是人,他们也应当享受权利与尊严,联合国大会将每年的 12 月 3 日作为"国际残疾人日"(International Day of Disabled Persons)。

二、护理人员学习残疾的意义

保障残疾人得到平等的对待,因为他们有相同的需要和相同的治疗权利。

需要了解如何有效地与有各种残疾的患者进行沟通,包括耳聋或听力较差的人,或有语言、视觉或智力残疾的人。

三、残疾分类

残疾分为 6 类:肢体残疾、视力残疾、听力残疾、智力残疾、学习障碍、精神障碍。

1. **肢体残疾** 可以是波动的或间歇性的、慢性的、渐进的或稳定的、可见的或不可见的。有些会带来极端的疼痛,有些不伴有疼痛感。

常见的渐进式身体残疾有慢性关节炎、多发性硬化症。常见的非渐进式身体残疾有脑瘫、脊柱裂。

2. **视力残疾** 由于各种原因使视觉器官或大脑视中枢的构造或功能发生部分或完全病变,导致双眼不同程度的视力损失或视野缩小,视功能难以像一般人一样在从事工作、学习或进行其他活动时应用自如,甚至丧失。只有 10% 的人是全盲,90% 的人有视力障碍。例如:色盲、白内障、青光眼。

3.听力残疾 由于各种原因导致双耳不同程度的永久性听力障碍,听不到或听不清周围环境声或言语声,以致影响日常生活和社会参与。残疾程度从听力障碍到严重的听力损失。

4.智力残疾 以认知发展和能力明显低于平均水平为特征,一个人的学习能力会受到永久的限制。

智力残疾产生的原因可能有:孕期母亲的疾病的影响、孕期间使用酒精或药物、遗传、儿童疾病。

5.学习障碍 学习障碍本质上是一个人的中枢神经系统的特定和持续的紊乱,影响学习过程。这影响一个人解读他们的所见所闻,或者将大脑不同部位的信息联系起来的能力。有学习障碍并不意味着一个人没有学习能力,而是他们以不同的方式学习。

6.精神障碍 精神障碍是指各类精神障碍持续1年以上未痊愈,存在认知、情感和行为障碍,影响日常生活和活动参与的状况。在精神残疾中,精神分裂症所占比例最大。精神障碍可以有多种形式,如抑郁症、焦虑症、神经性厌食症和暴食症、阿尔茨海默病、脑卒中、痴呆等。

四、导致残疾的主要原因

除了遗传因素造成的残疾外,还有很多后天的原因,主要有外伤(脑或脊髓损伤)、感染(脑炎)、接触有害物质(一氧化碳)、情绪剥夺或缺乏刺激、营养不良。

第二节 残疾的心理反应阶段

慢性疾病或残疾的发作通常会触发一系列的心理反应,分为6个阶段。

1.无知期 是指一个人患病后或者身体功能出现障碍后,对自己的真实病情并不了解,而且没有认识到病情的严重性,心理上没有一个长期应对病情和残障的准备。

2.震惊期 指患者听到或是意识到自己病情的严重程度后,在心理上出现的麻木或者休克的状态。震惊期一般出现在无知期之后,持续的时间从几秒到数天不等。

3.否认期 在经过震惊期打击后,患者为避免自己出现更大的精神痛苦,心理上否认已发生的事实。

4.抑郁期 患者在完全意识到自己病情的严重性及可能出现的结果后,心理防线彻底瓦解,对自己的疾病以及今后的生活评价多是负面的,持续处于抑郁的情绪状态。抑郁期持续时间一般为数月或更长时间。

5.反对独立期 是指患者经过抑郁期后,情绪已经趋于稳定,但是在行为上出现倒退,缺乏积极独立的谋生心态及行为。

6.适应期 患者经过以上阶段后,心理上对自己的病情及预后不再过分地担心,并能主动面对自己的疾病和以后的生活,积极地配合各种治疗,在心理上基本适应了因疾病给自己造成的不适。

护士必须了解残疾及残疾对人产生的影响,帮助患者,满足患者的需求,为残疾患者提供舒适和高质量的护理。

在护理过程中,护士作为患者的咨询师,提供情感、智力和心理支持,倾听他们,与他们建立融洽的治疗关系;作为患者的教育者,必要时提供足够的信息;作为患者的劝导者,帮助患者改变行为和生活方式;作为患者的倡导者,代表患者发言。

练习题

1. 国际残疾人日是(　　)
   A. 12 月 3 日　　　　B. 12 月 4 日　　　　C. 11 月 3 日　　　　D. 11 月 4 日

2. 以认知发展和能力明显低于平均水平为特征的,一个人的学习能力会受到永久的限制是(　　)
   A. 智力残疾　　　　B. 学习障碍　　　　C. 精神障碍　　　　D. 视力残疾

3. 导致残疾的主要原因,不包括(　　)
   A. 遗传因素　　　　B. 外伤(脑或脊髓损伤)　　C. 感染(脑炎)　　D. 情绪失控

4. 患者听到或是意识到自己病情的严重程度后,在心理上出现的麻木或者是休克的状态,是心理反应的(　　)
   A. 无知期　　　　B. 震惊期　　　　C. 否认期　　　　D. 抑郁期

5. 患者在完全意识到自己病情的严重性及可能出现的结果后,心理防线彻底瓦解是心理反应的(　　)
   A. 否认期　　　　B. 抑郁期　　　　C. 反对独立期　　　　D. 适应期

参考答案

第十八章 住院治疗

第一节 概　述

一、住院的定义

住院即患者住进医院接受治疗或观察。

二、心理护理的程序

1. 心理护理评估　心理护理评估是根据心理学的理论和方法对患者的心理状态进行全面、系统和深入的客观描述。护士在评估患者现存的或潜在的心理社会问题时,首先要收集信息,当发现问题存在于哪个范围时,可将评估聚焦于该范围,称为聚焦性评估。对刚入院的患者,初次心理护理评估应包括基本资料、患者对健康状况的感知、营养与代谢、排泄功能、意志活动水平、睡眠与休息、感知和认知、自我认知、角色关系、承受应激能力。

2. 心理护理诊断　心理护理诊断是在心理评估的基础上对所收集的资料进行分析,从而确定护理对象的心理健康问题及引起心理健康问题的原因,是护士为达到预期结果选择心理护理措施的基础。

3. 心理护理计划　心理护理计划是针对心理护理诊断提出的护理问题而制订的适用于个体的具体心理干预措施。计划的内容及步骤应包括:排列心理护理诊断的顺序;确定预期目标;制订心理护理措施;护理计划成文。

4. 心理护理实施　心理护理实施是指为实现心理护理目标,执行心理护理计划,解决护理对象心理问题的过程。所有提出的心理护理诊断都要通过实施各种心理护理措施来得到解决。

5. 心理护理评价　心理护理评价是对患者接受心理护理后产生的认知、情绪和行为变化的鉴定和判断。护理评价应贯穿整个心理护理的全过程,并应根据评估结果进行相应的调整。

第二节　不同年龄阶段住院患者的心理特点

一、儿童患者的心理特点

1. 分离性焦虑　　儿童住院治疗,离开了主要抚养人和熟悉的环境,首先会出现"分离性焦虑",表现为焦虑不安、经常哭闹、拒食、不服药、睡眠不安等,加之医院陌生的环境、其他儿童的哭闹,均会加重患儿的焦虑。

2. 恐惧、抗拒　　恐惧也是患儿的主要表现之一。患儿住院离开父母和熟悉的环境、对诊疗措施的不了解以及强迫接受一些诊疗措施,均会导致儿童出现恐惧情绪。在强烈的恐惧情绪影响之下,有的患儿会出现拒绝住院、拒绝接受治疗,或者大喊大叫、摔东西等表现;也有的患儿对前来探视的父母抗拒、不理睬,以此来表现自己不愉快的心情。

3. 皮肤饥饿　　人类与所有的热血动物一样,都有一种特殊的需要,即相互接触与抚摸,这种现象称为"皮肤饥饿"。亲子抚触是婴儿非常重要的心理需求,年龄较小的住院患儿,离开了母亲,这种特殊需要得不到满足,常表现为哭闹、食欲减退、睡眠不安等。

4. 行为退化　　疾病带来的痛苦和折磨,加之住院引起的焦虑、恐惧情绪,都可能导致患儿出现行为退化,如尿床、撒娇、拒食、睡前哭闹、被动依赖等。

二、青年患者的心理特点

青年人的心理特点是迅速走向成熟而又尚未成熟,这就决定了青年患者在面对疾病时情绪往往变化无常,具有明显的两极性,容易从一个极端走向另一个极端。

1. 震惊与否认　　青年人对人生和未来充满了无限的憧憬和向往。此时得知自己得病,尤其是重大疾病,首先会感到震惊,难以接受,进而不相信医生的诊断,出现"否认"的表现,否认自己得病,很难进入患者角色,拒绝接受治疗。直到真正感到病痛的折磨和体力虚弱时才逐渐接受患病的事实。

2. 焦虑与急躁　　青年人还常常担心疾病会给学习、工作、恋爱、结婚等带来不利影响,表现出焦虑不安。治疗中往往急于求成,缺乏耐心,希望能一蹴而就,一旦治疗达不到预期效果,或者出现病情反复,就表现出急躁情绪。病情有所好转时又往往盲目乐观,不按医嘱用药、不配合治疗。

3. 悲观与失望　　当疾病进入慢性期或留下后遗症甚至恶化时,会对青年人造成很大的打击,容易出现沮丧、悲观、失望甚至抑郁的情绪。青年人容易表现出极端心理和行为,自暴自弃,放弃治疗,甚至产生自杀的想法。

4. 孤独与寂寞　　青年人住院后,离开了熟悉的家庭、学校、同学和伙伴,住进陌生的医院,只能自己默默承受疾病的痛苦,过着单调、无趣的生活。住院时间稍长就会出现孤单、寂寞、无聊等情绪。

三、中年患者的心理特点

中年人在家庭和社会中都承担重要的角色,人格和情绪较稳定,但一旦生病,往往表现出复杂的心理活动。

1. 焦虑与急躁　　中年人由于其重要的家庭、社会角色,患病后更容易出现焦虑情绪。焦虑情绪又会导致其在疾病治疗时表现出急躁的情绪,进而不能安心养病,希望能尽快治愈,尽早出院。有的患者会因为种种原因而放弃自身的健康,中断治疗,提前出院。

2. 悲观与抑郁　中年人患病后不能正常工作,经济来源减少,加之昂贵的医疗费,以及赡养父母、子女教育等问题,使其产生悲观、失望的情绪,感到强烈的无助感和无望感,甚至产生轻生的念头,以此来减轻家庭的经济负担或者逃避其内心的煎熬。

3. 更年期综合征　中年人在体力和精力上开始向老年人过渡,常出现体力和精力不济的表现。此时患病,会加速这种转变,可出现更年期综合征,有明显的自主神经功能紊乱症状,如头痛、头晕、失眠、食欲减退、心悸、气短、畏寒、怕热等。

四、老年患者的心理特点

1. 自尊心强　老年人的自尊心比较强,希望得到医生、护士的尊重。不愿听从别人的安排,尤其不重视年轻医护人员的意见。有时甚至突然拒绝进行治疗和护理,有时又争强好胜,做一些力不能及的事情,如独自上厕所大小便、走路不用搀扶、坚持原有的饮食习惯,这样很容易导致一些意外的发生。

2. 自卑和抑郁　老年人社会地位和家庭地位的下降,以及身体的日渐衰弱,常常产生自卑心理。一旦生病,常感到自己在世的日子不长,许多想做的事情无法去完成,进一步加重自卑和无价值感。老年人多患慢性或老化性疾病,对疾病痊愈往往信心不足,自怨自艾,进而产生抑郁情绪,因此而自杀的老年人也并不少见。

3. 恐惧、孤独　当病情较重时,老年人常意识到死亡的来临,故表现出怕死、恐惧等情绪反应。这些情绪有的溢于言表,更多的则隐藏在心底。老年人害怕孤独,在患病时表现尤为突出,他们渴望得到别人的慰藉、照料、陪伴。

4. 以自我为中心　有些老年人性情刻板、固执,常常以自我为中心,生病住院后也常要求医护人员的诊疗工作要符合自己的生活秩序和习惯;也常常要求家人给予自己更多关注,对家人过度依赖。

5. 退化　有的老年人生病后情感和行为变得幼稚,常提出不切实际的要求,情绪波动大,自控能力差,常与家人、病友、医护人员发生冲突。有的老年人小病大养,不愿出院,对医护人员和家人依赖,自己能做的事情也需要别人帮助,甚至和小孩一样,出现"老小孩"现象。

6. 回避　部分老年患者患病后为避免精神上的压力,长期回避与疾病有关的事件或话题,在人前表现得若无其事而独处时常常落泪,深藏自己的内心感受。

第三节　情绪问题的心理护理

患者在患病后常出现的情绪问题主要有焦虑、抑郁、恐惧、愤怒。

一、焦虑

1. 焦虑的定义　焦虑是指患者在面临不够明确的、模糊的或即将出现的威胁或危险时,所感受到的一种不愉快的情绪体验。常见于以下患者:儿童或老年患者、新入院及新入监护室患者、手术患者以及其他进行特殊或有创的诊疗护理措施前的患者。

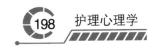

2.焦虑的心理护理

(1)建立良好的护患关系:建立良好的护患关系对心理护理的效果有重要影响,要求护士在实施心理护理过程中,始终把良好的护患关系放在头等重要位置,并贯穿心理护理过程的始终。

(2)提供适当的支持:护士能提供给患者的支持包括信息支持、情感支持和社会支持。信息支持是指患者所需要的各种知识,如医院的规章制度,疾病的诊断、治疗、预后等相关知识。

(3)心理咨询和治疗的技术:①放松疗法;②系统脱敏疗法;③生物反馈疗法;④理性情绪行为疗法。

(4)精神药物治疗:焦虑状况比较严重的患者,可以建议请精神科会诊,进行心理治疗或药物治疗。

二、抑郁

1.抑郁的定义 抑郁表现为情绪低落、思维迟钝、兴趣减退或丧失,因感到生活无意义、前途无望而郁郁寡欢,严重者甚至有自杀观念或自杀行为。身患重病、久治不愈和老年患者常出现抑郁情绪。

2.抑郁的心理护理 根据评估的结果和心理问题的层次,结合临床具体情况选择合适的心理护理技术对患者实施心理护理。

(1)良好的护患关系。

(2)积极寻求社会支持:鼓励患者多向亲人、朋友、医务人员倾诉,寻求更多社会支持。

(3)心理咨询和治疗的技术:①理性情绪行为疗法;②家庭治疗;③放松疗法;④催眠疗法。

(4)积极参加社会活动:当患者处于抑郁状态时,可以鼓励其在身体条件允许的情况下,多参加各种社会活动,以转移其对疾病和躯体症状的注意力。

(5)心理治疗或精神药物治疗:抑郁状况比较严重的患者,可以建议请精神科会诊,进行心理治疗或药物治疗。

三、恐惧

1.恐惧的定义 恐惧是患者面临某种具体而明确的威胁或危险时所产生的一种心理体验。临床上儿童和手术患者最常出现恐惧情绪。引起恐惧的因素有医院特殊的氛围和环境、疾病的威胁、一定危险性或有创性的检查、手术、预后不良或威胁生命的疾病等。

2.恐惧的心理护理

(1)消除恐惧的对象和原因:护士要分析并确认患者出现恐惧的原因和情境,护士应在患者恐惧之前,主动将可能给患者带来的痛苦和威胁作适当说明,以减弱或消除危险情境,并适当给予患者暗示和保证。

(2)心理咨询和治疗的技术:①示范法;②阳性强化法;③放松疗法;④理性情绪行为疗法;⑤系统脱敏疗法,帮助患者从恐惧等级较低的情境开始放松,直至其能面对最恐惧的情境;⑥宣泄。

四、愤怒

1.愤怒的定义 愤怒是个人需要不能得到满足,愿望不能实现,在追求某一目标的道路上遇到障碍、受到挫折时产生的情绪体验。

2.愤怒的心理护理 由于医疗行业的特殊性,医务人员工作中时常会遇到各种患者愤怒的情境。患者出现愤怒情绪不仅会降低其对治疗护理的配合及医务人员的信任,影响疾病的治疗,而且容易加深医患矛盾,引起医疗纠纷,严重损害医院和医务人员的形象。与愤怒患者实现有效沟通,实施良好的心理护理,在当今医疗环境下显得尤为重要。

（1）理解、接纳患者的愤怒情绪:问至少3句可能与诊疗核心情况无关的其他"看似废话"的问题,让患者能回答出"是的",让患者对护士的问话形成认同,如针对腹痛患者护士护理时可以问"您是否感觉到腹痛?""您希望尽快缓解疼痛吗?""您是否很着急?"这样的问话能使患者感觉被理解、被接纳,为实现进一步的沟通打下基础。

（2）改变环境:患者情绪稳定之后,找一个利于沟通的环境,如安静、舒适的办公室或会议室,脱离引起患者愤怒的情境和人物。同时也要做好自我保护措施,沟通环境中不能有能造成伤害的物件,如刀具、玻璃器械等;用固定不能移动的凳子,护士坐靠门边的位置。

（3）心理咨询和治疗的技术:①情绪宣泄,②支持性心理干预,③放松疗法。

练习题

1. 婴幼儿患病住院后最突出的心理反应是( )

A. 分离性焦虑　　　B. 思念亲人　　　　　　C. 恐惧

D. 皮肤饥饿　　　　E. 行为异常

2. 患者最常见、最重要的心理变化是( )

A. 人格变化　　　　B. 意志变化　　　　　　C. 情绪变化

D. 认知功能变化　　E. 以上都不是

3. 关于患者的心理描述,下列不正确的是( )

A. 进入患者角色后,对自身的注意力明显增强

B. 进入患者角色后,最常见、最突出的心理变化是情绪变化

C. 患者产生依赖心理和依赖行为是正常的心理反应

D. 患者的人格在疾病的影响下可以发生变化

E. 人格具有稳定性,即使疾病的影响也不会改变

4. 关于心理护理,下列说法正确的是( )

A. 心理护理是整体护理的核心部分　　　　B. 心理护理贯穿于整体护理的过程中

C. 心理护理就是做思想工作　　　　　　　D. 心理护理不限于互相交谈

E. 心理护理不同于心理治疗

5. 对焦虑患者进行护理,下列哪项措施不对( )

A. 首先要建立良好的护患关系,取得患者的信任　B. 帮助患者认识焦虑

C. 使用放松技术　　　　　　　　　　　　D. 一旦出现焦虑应给予抗焦虑药物

E. 以上都不对

6. 急危重症患者初入院的1~2d,最典型的心理特点是( )

A. 焦虑、恐惧　　　B. 否认　　　　　　　　C. 孤独、愤怒

D. 依赖　　　　　　E. 自我形象紊乱

7. 某神志清醒,正接受紧急救治的急性心肌梗死患者,目睹医护人员镇定自若的神情却依然圆睁双目、焦躁不安。此时该患者的最主要情绪反应可能是( )

A. 过度焦虑　　　　B. 严重抑郁　　　　　　C. 高度紧张

D. 极度恐慌　　　　E. 创伤应激综合征

8. "癌症患者的心理护理属于共性化心理护理"的说法( )

A. 正确　　　　　　B. 不确切　　　　　　　C. 有道理

D. 错误　　　　　　E. 以上均不当

9. 与患者的沟通中,老年患者最强烈的需要是(　　　)

A. 安全的需要　　　　B. 交往的需要　　　　C. 尊重的需要

D. 情感的需要　　　　E. 信息的需要

10. 患者不安心住院治疗,常见于(　　　)

A. 思念亲人的儿童患者　　　　　　　B. 挂念学业的青年患者

C. 工作繁忙或家庭责任重大的中年患者　　D. 担心家庭经济负担的老年患者

E. 以上都是

参考答案

第十九章　损失和哀伤

▓▓▓▓▓▓ **学习目标** ▓▓▓▓▓▓

1. 掌握损失定义。
2. 熟悉哀伤定义。
3. 了解损失和哀伤在医疗环境中的影响。

第一节　损　失

一、损失的定义

损失指失去某物或某人的事实或过程,当某人或某物不再被看到、听到、知道、感觉到或体验到时发生。

因死亡而失去亲人(丧亲)可能发生在生命周期的任何阶段(非常规性影响)。然而,随着年龄的增长,这种可能性变得更大。有些损失比其他损失更"不常规",例如失去孩子。这可能发生在从受孕到青春期及以后的任何阶段。流产、死产和新生儿死亡都是丧亲的形式,或被称作终止妊娠。

遭受丧亲之痛(无论采取何种形式)的人发生的心理和身体反应称为哀伤。"可观察到的哀伤表达"被称为哀悼,尽管这个词经常用于指代围绕死亡的社会习俗(例如葬礼和穿黑衣服)。

但是哀伤可以在实际死亡之前"开始",而那些正在死去的人也可以为自己的死亡而哀伤。护士在帮助绝症患者接受病情方面发挥着至关重要的作用。他们处于能够倾听患者谈论希望和恐惧的特殊地位,护士的经验、知识和技能可能使患者能够探索他们的感受并接受他们的病情。

损失示例见表19-1。

表 19-1　损失示例

损失	示例
熟悉的环境	地震
自我的一部分	身体部位缺失(截肢者)或功能丧失(听力损失)或自尊受损(被雇主解雇)

续表 19-1

损失	示例
独立	入狱
关系	离婚
财务安全	破产
社会地位	成为难民
爱的人或事物	父母或宠物去世

二、损失的类型

1. 突然损失　意外事故、心脏病发作。
2. 逐渐损失　疾病逐渐恶化、老去和慢性疾病迁延不愈。
3. 预期损失　预期和可预测的损失进展。
4. 不确定损失　某些疾病具有高度不确定性(传染病)。
5. 重大损失　亲人去世、绝症。
6. 部分损失　带走一部分身体的疾病和残疾,例如乳房切除术。
7. 永久损失　没有康复的希望,例如肾衰竭。
8. 暂时损失　有希望康复的,例如腺瘤。

第二节　哀　伤

一、哀伤的定义

哀伤是对损失的自然反应。哀伤是一种正常的反应,可以帮助一个人从损失中慢慢恢复。在临终前为临终者悲痛的过程(预期性哀伤)是一个"放手"的过程。

哀伤被描述为:一种人类的自然反应,一种精神紊乱,一种疾病的过程。

这三种描述方法都包含事实的一部分。就第一种而言,哀伤是人类存在的普遍特征,在所有文化中都可以找到。但它的形式和表达的强度差别很大。就第二种而言,尽管哀伤本身从未被归类为精神障碍,但精神病学框架强调了哀伤所涉及的人类痛苦,因此提供了一个有用的平衡,将其简单地视为一种自然反应。关于第三种,虽然丧亲者的发病率(健康恶化)或死亡率(死亡)可能会增加,但这些不一定是由哀伤过程直接引起的。例如,生活方式改变(如改变营养或药物摄入)的影响,或在丧亲之前增加对身体疾病的关注,可能会被误认为是哀伤本身的影响。然而,有大量证据表明,与匹配的非失去亲人的对照组相比,失去亲人的夫妻更有可能死亡。这主要适用于鳏夫,尤其是经历意外丧亲的年轻鳏夫。

急性哀伤是在损失时开始的反应,例如因事故而失去肢体。并非所有人都以完全相同的方式哀伤,哀伤的时间长短各不相同。

二、哀伤的类型

1. 预期　在实际损失之前。例如,对于家庭中照顾临终亲人的人来说,哀伤可能在临终亲人去世之前很久就开始了。

2. 急性　在损失时。

3. 慢性　持续较长时间且可能是间歇性的哀伤。例如,残疾的孩子的父母。

4. 延迟　推迟到以后的时间。例如,妻子因为需要先照顾孩子而推迟对丈夫的死亡的哀伤。

5. 压抑　被压抑/克制多年,需要触发因素。例如,一位母亲流产了,但压抑了自己的哀伤,后来在自己的女儿流产时才过分地表现出来。

三、哀伤的阶段

每个人都不一定要经历所有的阶段,也不一定要按任何精确的顺序经历这些阶段。

库伯勒·罗斯的阶段理论描述基于她对200多名绝症患者的开创性工作。她对患者如何为即将到来的死亡(预期哀伤)做准备很感兴趣,因此她的阶段理论描述了临终的过程。她受到了早期的鲍尔比理论的启发,她的阶段理论后来被其他研究人员应用。她的理论在护理和心理咨询方面非常有影响力,包括针对临终的患者和失去亲人的人。

1. 第一个阶段为否认和自我孤立　这个阶段伴随着诸如"这不可能发生在我身上、这不是真的"之类的想法。在情感上否认已经发生或即将发生的损失。患者通常退出社交活动,可能会寻求另外几位医生的意见,希望最初的诊断是不正确的。这可以防止患者因最初的震惊而不知所措。大多数患者不仅在他们疾病的早期阶段使用否认(或至少部分否认),而且在以后也会使用。就好像他们可以在一定的时间段内考虑自己死亡的可能性,但随后必须摆脱这种想法,以便他们可以继续生活。否认充当一个缓冲机制,让患者有时间发展其他应对机制。它也可以带来孤立。患者可能害怕在痛苦中被拒绝和抛弃,认为没有人了解痛苦是什么样的。无论出于何种原因,医护人员的回避都会加剧绝症患者的这种孤立感。

库伯勒·罗斯采访的几乎所有患者最初都否认他们患有危及生命的疾病,只有3个人一直处于否认状态(其余的人摇摆不定)。当某人以突然或冷漠的方式得到诊断时,或者如果他们被家人和(或)同样否认的工作人员包围时,否认更为常见。寻求第二个意见是一个非常普遍的初始反应,代表了一种绝望的尝试,以改变他们刚刚被推入到的不可预测的世界,回到他们所知道和理解的世界。

2. 第二个阶段为愤怒　开始意识到损失并体验到诸如"为什么是我? 为什么会发生这种情况? 为什么是现在?"这样的想法。当他开始意识到无法改变现状时,他可能会感到愤怒和沮丧。这可能是针对医生、护士、亲戚,其他继续生活的健康人。这可能是家人和护理人员最难应对的阶段,他们可能会对患者的愤怒做出反应,并以自己的愤怒做出回应,这只会增加患者的敌对行为。

3. 第三个阶段为讨价还价　当人们试图通过达成"交易"来推迟现实时发生,例如,渴求与命运做交易。这是通过与命运(或医院)"做交易"来推迟死亡的尝试,就像孩子为了自己的要求可能与父母讨价还价一样。因此,它必须包括一个"良好行为"奖,并设定一个自我强加的"截止日期",例如儿子或女儿的婚礼。患者承诺,如果批准死亡的延期,则不会要求更多生存时间。

4. 第四个阶段为沮丧　当患者开始意识到无法改变现状时,他可能会感到沮丧。他为死亡所代表的所有损失而哀伤。这是预备性抑郁,一种预期性哀伤,这种情感帮助患者为最终与世界分离做好准备。反应性抑郁症包括恐惧和焦虑的表达以及对身体形象、工作、经济保障或继续照顾孩子的能力的巨大损失感。抑郁是临终者的常见反应。例如辛顿说,18%的自杀者患有严重的身体疾病,其中的4%患有可能会在6个月内导致他们死亡的疾病。过着充实生活的老年人相对来说没有什么可悲哀的——他们获得了很多,失去的很少。但矛盾的是,那些认为生活充满错误和错失机会的人可能会更加悲痛,因为他们开始意识到这些机会现在已经永远失去了。这类似于埃里克森理论中的绝望,就像库伯勒·罗斯将其与接受区别开来一样。达到接受阶段的人的超然和平静来自冷静,而那些否认阶段的人则充满绝望。后者不能接受死亡,也不能再否认它的存在。库伯勒·罗斯发现只有少数患者会战斗到最后,挣扎并保持希望,这使得他们几乎不可能真正地到达接受阶段。

5. 第五个阶段为接受　即可能会意识到情况的必然性并接受损失。他对自己的命运感到沮丧或愤怒,并且能够谈论他的损失。患者几乎剥离了任何感受,似乎放弃了生命的挣扎,睡得更多,远离他人,仿佛在为"长途旅行"做准备。希望(对于治愈或奇迹)是贯穿所有这些阶段的持续线索,对于在疾病中保持患者的精神面貌是必要的。希望对某些人来说是痛苦的合理化,对另一些人来说是一种急需的否认方式。罗斯发现,如果患者停止表达希望,通常是即将死亡的迹象。

四、帮助哀伤的人

完全没有哀伤、不健康的迹象和未解决的哀伤会导致延迟或扭曲的反应。哀伤的人可能会经历多种感受:震惊、愤怒、哀伤、内疚、沮丧、绝望、解脱、希望和接受。情绪表达可能包括:哭泣、远离人群、缺乏活力、没有动力、敌对行为、身体症状(例如无法入睡、无法进食、胸痛、头痛、肠胃不适)。

医护人员必须允许并鼓励患者克服哀伤,通过倾听来表达感受。根据马奇的说法,大多数护士经常面对死亡的现实,这些经历会令一般人感到震惊……死亡是一场重大危机,它可能令人痛苦、陌生和恐惧。为了帮助患者和他们的家人度过这个过程,护士需要培养自己面对绝症和死亡的态度和能力。

第三节　在医疗环境中的损失和悲伤

一、与临终的成年患者交流

研究表明,一部分临终患者不希望谈论他们病情的严重性。他们通过避免专注于治疗预期或在令人轻松愉快的谈话中寻求逃避来应对死亡。尽管如此,研究者们仍然建议护士把与患者讨论他们对预后的感受作为通用的规则来遵守。

迪恩建议护士培养沟通技巧,这不仅能让他们能够感性地与患者谈论临终和死亡,而且让他们有能力评估患者是否想要去进行讨论。同样,帕金森认为,提供与患者交谈的机会以便让患者表达恐惧、愤怒或抑郁应该是护士工作的主要重点。

韦伯斯特观察到在4家英国医院的护士与临终的患者交流中,护士经常表现出"阻碍"的行为,他们通过改变话题、忽视暗示、开玩笑或用避重就轻的方式来调整他们的反应来避免亲密和深入的对话。这种轻松愉快的互动使护士能够回避潜在的困难对话,使他们与患者之间保持在情感上的"安全地带"。威尔金森在54名癌症护士身上观察到了类似的行为,他们表现出的阻碍行为大大多于促进行为。例如,在观察到的护患交流过程中,从未讨论过妇科、膀胱或肠道恶性肿瘤可能对患者生活产生的性心理影响。科斯特洛证实了这一点。

根据黑尔和普拉特的说法,直到现在,病房里的死亡仍然是对护理或医学上的失败的强烈暗示。但医疗上的重大发展,例如临终关怀运动的发展,表明医疗的重点正在从治疗患者转向关怀患者。马齐坚持认为,"护理正在被重新定义,去涵盖全心全意地照顾临终患者或失去亲人的人……"自1960年以来,西方文化普遍朝着关于死亡和临终的公开交流迈进,家长式的观念,即认为患者会因为太沮丧而无法讨论死亡的观念正在慢慢改变。

二、与临终的患儿交流

即使没有被明确告知,患有危及生命的疾病的儿童仍能够感觉到他们的病情很严重,知道他们可能会死去或即将死去。即使接受相同数量和持续时间的治疗,他们的焦虑水平也明显高于慢性病儿童。当孩子不在医院时,例如在白血病儿童疾病缓解期间,这种焦虑和孤立感仍然存在。

当另一个孩子在病房里死去时,住院临终的孩子对死亡的意识会更加集中。如果孩子患有同样的疾病,那么该事件与临终的孩子即将死亡之间的联系就会更加直接。贾德认为,大多数医院在儿童病房对于临终患儿的态度更加开放和诚实,有时会与孩子公开讨论死亡和临终问题,这具体取决于该医疗机构的道德准则。

与临终患儿的有效沟通受到护士的价值观、态度和信仰的影响,而这些价值观、态度和信仰反过来又受到过去的经验以及宗教、文化和社会信仰的影响。研究表明,医生和护士在保持距离和疏远方面表现得很熟练。这些策略可能有助于保护医疗从业者免受痛苦,但也会阻碍与临终患儿的有效沟通。有的家庭可能不希望公开讨论孩子即将死亡的事情,以保护孩子免受痛苦或是因为家人自己的恐惧。这种"相互伪装"——库伯勒·罗斯提出的相互伪装意识被证明在维持希望和家庭成员的角色方面发挥着重要的作用。

显然,临终的患儿需要一个适合其年龄和发育的机会来分享恐惧和担忧。这并不意味着要强加对临终话题的讨论,而是需要对患儿的谈话意愿(或其他表达方式)持开放态度。如果患儿似乎在情感上"心不在焉",但没有抑郁,这可能是一种非常容易理解的与周围世界分离的方式。这应该是被容忍和尊重的,而不是为了患儿或家人而强迫患儿快乐或"坚持"。正如贾德所指出的,这种选择撤离的方式可能是患儿所剩的唯一可以掌控自己的方式。

三、急诊科中的死亡

死亡的消息会引起人们警觉:世界突然变成一个充满威胁的、不可预测的地方。任何使损失变得不真实的事情,例如突然的、意外的死亡和发生在不寻常或暴力情况下的死亡,都可能使其更难以接受,这可能会产生更持久和更复杂的悲伤反应。与在其他领域工作的护士相比,急诊科护士可能需要处理更高比例的此类死亡。事实上,1/3的医院死亡发生在患者到达后的最初几个小时内。

根据史密斯的说法,尽管临终关怀和姑息治疗运动在帮助护士和患者做好准备迎接死亡和癌症、艾滋病等疾病的终末期方面起了巨大的作用,但许多急症护理护士仍然感到毫无准备和缺乏支持。我们生活在一个心血管疾病和意外事故是导致死亡的主要原因的社会中,而这些死亡往往发生在医院里,对医护人员的预先警告很少或根本没有,更不用说对于亲戚或朋友了。

赖特研究了美国急诊室(以及ICU、CCU和儿科ICU)中护士应对突发死亡的问题。他得出的结论是,患者亲属和医院工作人员的心理健康状态取决于患者到达急诊室之前所打下的基础。他现在在英国经营危机培训、教育和咨询(CRI-TEC),为受突发死亡影响的人提供支持服务。该机构为卫生专业人员、警察和消防队提供课程。

对刚失去亲人的患者家属来说,心理健康人员应该能够及早提供支持,这可以为亲属的康复过程提供基础保障。但护理人员和医务人员常常感到准备不足,无法满足亲属的需求。在急诊科中,由于医疗工作人员和亲属在危机时刻见面,情况通常是复杂的,而交谈通常是短暂的、出乎意料的,

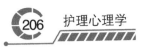

并且双方可能没有任何后续的接触。相比之下,病房环境通常允许有时间发展和融洽关系。急诊科的精神是拯救生命,因此当患者死亡时,这通常会导致医护人员有失败的感觉。但是,通过训练有素、积极主动的护理和医务人员的投入,能让他们了解对丧亲家属提供心理帮助的重要性,这可以帮助亲属的心理恢复。

练习题

1. 当某人或某物不再被看到、听到、知道、感觉到或体验到时发生,叫作(　　　)
   A. 损失　　　　　　　B. 死亡　　　　　　　C. 残疾　　　　　　　D. 悲伤

2. 遭受丧亲之痛的人发生的心理和身体反应被称为(　　　)
   A. 呆滞　　　　　　　B. 抑郁　　　　　　　C. 焦虑　　　　　　　D. 哀伤

3. 损失的类型不包括(　　　)
   A. 突然损失　　　　　B. 逐渐损失　　　　　C. 预期损失　　　　　D. 确定损失

4. 关于哀伤的定义,下列表述不正确的是(　　　)
   A. 一种社会反应　　　B. 一种人类的自然反应　　　C. 一种精神紊乱　　　D. 一种疾病的过程

5. 库伯勒·罗斯认为悲伤过程不包括(　　　)
   A. 否认　　　　　　　B. 悲伤　　　　　　　C. 讨价还价　　　　　D. 接受

6. 患者,男,63岁,肺癌晚期,身心非常痛苦,表现为悲伤、消沉、无望。此患者对其疾病的心理反应属于(　　　)
   A. 否认阶段　　　　　B. 愤怒阶段　　　　　C. 讨价还价阶段　　　D. 沮丧阶段

7. 哀伤的五个阶段中,最后一个阶段是(　　　)
   A. 否认阶段　　　　　B. 愤怒阶段　　　　　C. 讨价还价阶段　　　D. 接受阶段

8. 一位母亲流产了,但压抑了自己的哀伤,在后来自己的女儿流产时才表现出来,这属于(　　　)
   A. 预期的哀伤　　　　B. 急性的哀伤　　　　C. 慢性的哀伤　　　　D. 压抑的哀伤

9. 完全没有哀伤或不健康的迹象是一种正常的对损失的反应(　　　)
   A. 正确　　　　　　　B. 错误

10. 医护人员必须允许并鼓励患者克服哀伤,通过倾听来表达感受(　　　)
    A. 正确　　　　　　　B. 错误

参考答案

第二十章　临终护理

第一节　濒死和死亡

一、概念

1. **濒死的定义**　濒死即临终。指患者已经接受治疗性和姑息性的治疗后,虽然意识清楚,但病情加速恶化,各种迹象显示生命即将终结。因此濒死是生命活动的最后阶段。

2. **死亡的定义**　死亡是机体完整性的解体,是体内新陈代谢过程的停止,即是人生命活动的结束,也就是指个体的生命功能的永久终止。

二、死亡标准

1. **传统死亡标准**　将心跳、呼吸停止作为判断死亡的标准已经沿袭数千年。

2. **脑死亡标准**　目前医学界人士提出新的比较客观的标准,这就是脑死亡标准。脑死亡即全脑死亡,包括大脑、中脑、小脑和脑干的不可逆死亡。不可逆的脑死亡是生命活动结束的象征。1968年美国哈佛大学提出的脑死亡标准如下:①无感受性及反应性;②无运动、无呼吸;③无反射;④脑电波平坦。

上述标准须 24 h 内反复复查无改变,并排除体温低于 32 ℃ 及中枢神经抑制剂的影响,即可做出脑死亡的诊断。

三、死亡过程的分期

死亡不是骤然发生的,而是一个逐渐进展的过程,一般可分为 3 期。

1. **濒死期**　又称临终状态,是死亡过程的开始阶段。此期机体各系统的功能极度衰弱,中枢神经系统脑干以上部位的功能处于深度抑制状态,表现意识模糊或丧失,各种反射减弱或迟钝,肌张力减退或消失,心跳减弱,血压下降,呼吸微弱或出现潮式呼吸及间断呼吸。濒死期的持续时间可

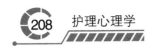

随患者机体状况及死亡原因而异,猝死等患者可直接进入临床死亡期。此期生命处于可逆阶段,及时有效的抢救治疗,生命可复苏;反之,则进入临床死亡期。

2. 临床死亡期　此期中枢神经系统的抑制过程已由大脑皮质扩散到皮质下部位,延髓处于极度抑制状态。表现为心跳、呼吸完全停止,瞳孔散大,各种反射消失,但各种组织细胞仍有微弱而短暂的代谢活动。此期一般持续 5~6 min,超过这个时限,大脑将发生不可逆的变化。但在低温条件下,尤其是头部降温,脑耗氧降低时,临床死亡期可延长达 1 h 或更久。

3. 生物学死亡期　生物学死亡期是死亡过程的最后阶段。此期整个中枢神经系统及各器官的新陈代谢相继停止,并出现不可逆的变化,整个机体已不可能复活。随着此期的进展,相继出现早期尸体现象,即尸冷、尸斑、尸僵等;晚期尸体现象,即尸体腐败等。

第二节　临终关怀

一、概念

临终关怀又称善终服务、安宁照顾、安息所等。临终关怀是向临终患者及家属提供一种全面的照料,包括生理、心理、社会等方面,使临终患者的生命得到尊重,症状得到控制,生命质量得到提高,家属的心身健康得到维护和增强,使患者在临终时能够无痛苦、安宁、舒适地走完人生的最后旅程。

二、临终关怀的发展

现代临终关怀创建于 20 世纪 60 年代,创始人桑得斯博士 1976 年在英国创办了世界第一所"圣克里斯多弗临终关怀医院",被誉为"点燃了世界临终关怀运动的灯塔"。从此以后美国、法国、日本、加拿大等 60 多个国家相继出现临终关怀服务。1988 年 7 月我国天津医学院在美籍华人黄天中博士的资助下,成立了中国第一个临终关怀研究中心,同年 10 月上海诞生了中国第一家临终关怀医院——南汇护理院。这些都标志着我国已跻身于世界临终关怀研究与实践的行列。之后,沈阳、北京、南京等多地都相继开展临终关怀服务,建立临终关怀机构。

三、临终关怀的研究对象

临终关怀不仅是一种服务,而且也是一门以探讨临终患者的生理、心理发展和为临终患者提供全面照料,减轻患者家属精神压力为研究对象,与医学、护理学、社会学、心理学、伦理学、卫生经济学、政策学、法学等多种学科领域密切相关的新兴边缘学科。

四、临终关怀的组织形式和理念

1. 临终关怀的组织形式　①临终关怀专门机构;②综合性医院内附设临终关怀病房;③居家照料。

2. 临终关怀的理念

(1)以治愈为主的治疗转变为以对症为主的照料:临终关怀是针对各种疾病的末期,治疗不再生效,生命即将结束者。对这些患者不是通过治疗使其免于死亡,而是通过全面的身心照料,提供给临终患者适度的、姑息性治疗,控制症状,解除痛苦,消除焦虑、恐惧,获得心理、社会支持,使其得到最后安宁。

（2）以延长患者的生存时间转变为提高患者的生命质量:临终关怀不以延长生存时间为重点,而以丰富患者有限生命,提高其临终阶段生命质量为宗旨,提供临终患者一个安适、有意义、有尊严、有希望的生活,让患者在有限的时间里,能有清醒的头脑,在可控制的病痛中,接受关怀,享受人生的最后旅途。

（3）尊重临终患者的尊严和权利:临终患者是临近死亡而尚未死亡者,只要他没有进入昏迷状态,就仍有思维、意识、情感,仍有人的尊严和权利。医护人员应注意维护和保持患者的价值和尊严,在临终照料中应允许患者保留原有的生活方式,尽量满足其合理要求,保留个人隐私权利,参与医护方案的制订等。

（4）注重临终患者家属的心理支持:在对临终患者全面照料的同时,也提供给临终患者家属心理、社会支持,从而使其获得接受亲人死亡事实的力量,坦然地面对亲人死亡。帮助患者家属既为患者生前提供服务,也为其死后提供居丧服务。

第三节　临终患者的生理变化及护理

一、生理变化

1. 感知觉、意识改变　表现为视觉逐渐减退直到视力消失。眼睑干燥,分泌物增多,瞳孔放大。听觉常常是人体最后消失的一个感觉。意识改变可表现为嗜睡、意识模糊、昏睡、昏迷等。

2. 肌肉张力丧失　表现为尿、便失禁,吞咽困难,无法维持良好舒适的功能体位,肢体软弱无力,不能进行自主躯体活动。脸部外观改变呈希氏面容,即面肌稍瘦、面部呈铅灰色、眼眶凹陷、双眼半睁、下颌下垂、嘴微张等。

3. 胃肠道蠕动逐渐减弱　表现为食欲减退、腹胀、恶心、呕吐、便秘、脱水、口干等。

4. 循环能力减退　表现为皮肤苍白、湿冷、大量出汗,四肢发绀、斑点,脉搏快而弱、不规则或测不出,血压降低或测不出,心尖搏动常最后消失。

5. 呼吸功能减退　表现为呼吸频率由快变慢,呼吸深度由深变浅,出现鼻翼呼吸、潮式呼吸、张口呼吸等,最终呼吸停止。可出现痰鸣音及鼾声呼吸。

6. 疼痛　表现为烦躁不安,血压及心率改变,呼吸变快或减慢,不寻常的姿势,疼痛面容,如五官扭曲、眉头紧锁、眼睛睁大或紧闭、双眼无神、咬牙等。

7. 临近死亡的体征　各种反射逐渐消失,肌张力减退、丧失,脉搏快而弱,血压降低,呼吸急促、困难,出现潮式呼吸,皮肤湿冷。通常呼吸先停止,随后心跳停止。猝死患者常心跳先停止。

二、护理措施

1. 促进患者舒适
（1）维持良好、舒适的体位,加强皮肤护理。
（2）重视口腔护理,晨起、餐后、睡前协助患者漱口,保持口腔清洁卫生。

2.营养支持

(1)主动向患者和家属解释出现消化系统症状的原因,以减少焦虑。

(2)注意食物的色、香、味,少量多餐,以减轻恶心,增进食欲。

(3)给予流质或半流质等便于患者吞咽的饮食。必要时采用鼻饲法或完全胃肠外营养,保证患者营养供给。

(4)加强监测,观察患者电解质指标及营养状况。

3.促进血液循环

(1)观察患者生命体征、皮肤颜色和温度。

(2)患者四肢冰冷不适时,应加强保暖,必要时给予热水袋,但水温不宜超过50 ℃。

(3)注意皮肤清洁、干燥。

4.改善呼吸功能

(1)保持室内空气新鲜,定时通风换气。

(2)神志清醒者,采用半卧位以扩大胸腔容量,减少回心血量,改善呼吸困难。昏迷者,采用仰卧位头偏向一侧或侧卧位,防止呼吸道分泌物误入气管引起窒息或肺部并发症。

(3)必要时使用吸引器吸出痰液,保持呼吸道通畅。

(4)视呼吸困难程度给予吸氧,纠正缺氧状态,改善呼吸功能。

5.减轻感觉与知觉刺激

(1)提供安静、空气新鲜、通风良好、有一定的保暖设施、适当的照明的环境,避免因患者视觉模糊产生害怕、恐惧心理,增加安全感。

(2)及时用湿纱布拭去眼部分泌物,患者眼睑不能闭合时可涂金霉素等眼药膏或覆盖凡士林纱布,以保护角膜,防止角膜干燥发生溃疡或结膜炎。

(3)护理中应防止在患者周围窃窃私语,以免增加患者的焦虑。可采用触摸患者等非语言交流方式,配合温和的语言。

练习题

1.现代医学已开始以下列哪项作为死亡的判断标准(　　　)

　　A.心跳停止　　　　　　　　B.呼吸停止　　　　　　　　C.脑死亡

　　D.心电图平直　　　　　　　E.瞳孔散大

2.死亡过程的第二期是(　　　)

　　A.临床死亡期　　　　　　　B.濒死期　　　　　　　　　C.否认期

　　D.生物学死亡期　　　　　　E.接受期

3.尸斑出现在死亡后(　　　)

　　A.2～4 h　　　　　　　　　B.2～6 h　　　　　　　　　C.4～6 h

　　D.6～8 h　　　　　　　　　E.7～8 h

4.临床死亡期指征不包括(　　　)

　　A.呼吸停止　　　　　　　　B.心跳停止　　　　　　　　C.各种反射消失

　　D.出现尸冷　　　　　　　　E.瞳孔散大

5.尸斑出现的部位是(　　　)

　　A.头顶部　　　　　　　　　B.面部　　　　　　　　　　C.腹部

　　D.胸部　　　　　　　　　　E.最低部位

6. 现代的临终关怀始于20世纪60年代,其创始人是( )
   A. 桑巴斯   C. 路易斯   B. 桑德斯
   D. 黄天中   E. 崔以泰

7. 中国第一个临终关怀研究中心成立于( )
   A. 上海   B. 广州   C. 天津
   D. 北京   E. 四川

8. 临终患者最后消失的感觉是( )
   A. 视觉   B. 听觉   C. 触觉
   D. 嗅觉   E. 味觉

9. 李女士,55岁,脑癌。入院时身体虚弱,接受抗癌治疗效果差。患者情绪不稳定,经常生气、愤怒、抱怨、与家属争吵。该期心理反应为( )
   A. 忧郁期   B. 愤怒期   C. 否认期
   D. 接受期   E. 协议期

10. 王先生,69岁,诊断为肝癌。病情日趋恶化,患者出现悲哀、情绪低落,要求见一些亲朋好友,并急于交代后事。此时患者心理反应属于( )
   A. 忧郁期   B. 愤怒期   C. 协议期
   D. 接受期   E. 否认期

参考答案

第二十一章　压力管理

▨▨▨▨▨▨▨▨ 学习目标 ▨▨▨▨▨▨▨▨

1. 掌握压力、压力源的含义。
2. 熟悉不同种类的压力源。
3. 了解压力对身体的影响，学习应对压力的方法。

第一节　压力的概述及压力事件

一、压力的概述

(一)压力的含义

压力指导致个体身体、情绪或心理紧张的任何类型的变化。任何的生活变动或习惯改变皆可称为压力。它是身体对任何需要注意或行动的事物的反应。

(二)压力源

1. 任何导致压力和减轻压力的因素　例如：来自情绪、身体、社会或经济方面的变化。

2. 准确识别压力源　有助于预测压力，大多数人在有准备的情况下能够更有效地应对压力事件。

(三)影响压力的因素

1. 压力源的性质　从大的方面讲，战争、地震、水灾、火灾等灾害，会给人们带来沉重的心理压力和负担。从小的方面讲，面临一次考试或考核、自己生病或亲友生病，也会给我们正常的生活带来意外的冲击和干扰，也都会成为我们心理压力的来源。在我们的生活中，压力如影随形地陪伴着我们，已成为我们生活的一部分。完全没有压力的情况是不存在的；换一种说法就是，没有压力本身就是一种压力，它的名字叫做空虚。

2. 压力源的数量　简单来说，个体在同一时间或一段时间内连续遭受的压力事件越多，压力就越大，反之亦然。

3. 持续时间　压力事件持续的时间越长，个体感受到的压力越大，反之亦然。

4. 可预测性　压力和压力事件的可预测性相关，如果个体能够很好地预测压力事件的发展方向，其感受到的压力就可能减小。

5. 严重程度　一般来说，压力过大时，人的理智一般难以控制，个体常表现出两种极端的行为反应,要么呆若木鸡,完全停止行动,要么兴奋激越,突然暴起攻击。中度心理压力一般会使人的行为能力降低,产生重复和刻板动作。在适度压力或轻度压力状况下,个体可能在理智控制下,充分发挥主观能动作用,对压力事件较妥善处理,从而也使自己心理承受力得到增强,动力性也随之增长。

6.应对方式　压力是一种主观反映,压力的大小,即人们不适应的心理感觉强度,它是由压力源事件的客观性和自我感觉的主观性两种因素共同决定的。在这两个重要因素中,起主导作用的还是人们的主观态度。可以说压力的大小,它是百分百听人们自己的,自己说它大,它就大;自己说它不大,它就不大;自己说没有,它就没有。用公式表达:压力的大小=压力源/承受力。

7.社会支持系统　压力之下,个体能够依靠自己的力量拨云见日最好,如果不能,就要积极地寻求社会支持和帮助。当个人遭遇重大压力与挫折而一时难以决策和承受时,应当优先运用咨询、求助策略,以使问题得以适当解决,建立由家人、朋友、同学、同事组成的网络危机干预组。机构组成的社会支持系统是提升压力与挫折应对能力的重要途径。

二、常见的压力事件

1.来自家庭的压力　包括复杂的亲情关系、子女成长问题、婚姻恋爱关系、家庭发展问题、家庭成员的重大事件等。

2.来自心理的压力　包括生理需要、安全需要、归属需要、尊重需要、自我实现需要等。

3.来自生理的压力　包括身体健康问题、个人形象问题等。

4.来自社会的压力　包括战争、天灾、人祸、社会的快速发展变化、各行业的竞争、人际关系的处理、挫折、冲突、生活变化等。

第二节　压力的反应及损害

一、压力的反应

1.躯体反应　个体在遭遇压力时,肾上腺髓质和肾上腺皮质被激活,肾上腺髓质引发短期应激反应,并分泌肾上腺素和去甲肾上腺素,最终引起一系列生理反应。例如:血糖升高、血管收缩、心跳加快、血液迅速从重要器官转移到心脏和骨骼肌并导致消化系统活动量减少、身体代谢率增加、细支气管扩张;肾上腺皮质引发长期应激反应,并分泌类固醇激素,非皮质激素通过肾脏滞留钠和水,增加血容量和血压,蛋白质和脂肪转化为葡萄糖或分解酶,降低能量需求,降低了身体免疫系统的反应。

2.心理反应　产生心理压力,精神紧张,难以放松。常见反应有无聊、空虚、持久的恐惧或忧虑、易怒、抱怨、自相矛盾、挫折感和攻击倾向、注意力不集中、动作迟缓、黯然神伤、心神不宁、疑心重重、优柔寡断、社交困难、麻木不仁、厌世、无精打采、崩溃感、濒死感等。

3.一般适应综合征　一般适应综合征为加拿大心理学家汉斯·薛利于1930年代提出,他认为这是个体为应对压力而产生的一类适应性反应:即一个有机体必须寻回他的平衡或稳定,从而维持或恢复其完整和安宁,未能应对或适应压力可能会产生"适应疾病",即溃疡、高血压和心脏病发作等。

一般适应综合征共包含3个阶段——警戒、抵抗和疲劳。

第一阶段,警戒阶段。当机体一旦接触到压力源时,就会调动能量来应对压力源的需要,并在躯体上表现出心跳加快、呼吸急促、出冷汗等一系列特定变化。这表明你的身体已经为立刻行动,如自卫或者夺路而逃做好了准备,但是如果刺激过强,则有可能导致机体的死亡。

第二阶段,抵抗阶段。如果压力源长时间没有被消除,机体就要长期面对压力源的存在。在此情况下,为了保持内在的平衡,机体需要转移到另外一种更为复杂的状态和水平从而来适应刺激。这种反应使机体的各种器官和腺体产生各种激素、盐、糖来给满足刺激所需要的能量,并保持身体的内部平衡。这时,警戒反应的特有指标会消失,而机体的各种反应将超出正常水平。

第三阶段,疲劳阶段。长时间的同样压力源之后,机体逐渐适应,而适应所需要的能量也随之消耗殆尽。警戒反应的特有指标再次出现。而现在的状态却是不可能挽回的。当机体不再能够抵抗施加在身上的压力源时就会崩溃、衰竭,并最终导致机体死亡(图21-1)。

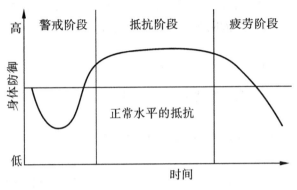

图21-1　一般适应综合征的时间阶段

二、压力对人体的危害

1. 生理方面　一个人压力过大的时候,最明显的反应就是肌肉紧张、心跳加快、血压升高、出汗等症状。医学家们发现,当人体压力过大时,会严重地影响人体的神经、骨骼、呼吸、心血管、内分泌、消化、生殖七大系统的健康。同时压力大还会引起过敏、头痛、心脏病等疾病的发生。

2. 心理方面　压力过大会造成注意力不集中,记忆力下降,理解力、创造力下降;经常担忧,烦躁不安,焦虑;产生神经质似的心理障碍,严重的甚至会出现感情淡漠、妄想、幻觉、自杀意念等病态心理现象。

3. 情绪方面　过大的压力让人产生不快乐、抑郁、焦虑、痛苦、不满、悲观以及闷闷不乐、反应过度的感觉,觉得生活毫无情趣,自制力下降,突然发怒、流泪或是大笑,独立工作能力下降。此外,压力大也容易使人变得健忘、倦怠、效率降低。再者,心理压力过大的人会变得冷漠而轻率。

4. 行为方面　压力过大会使人产生消极怠工、工作效率下降、逃避责任的反应;压力过大容易使人与他人发生冲突,人际关系恶化;压力过大会使人生活习惯改变,例如嗜烟、酗酒,甚至吸毒来麻痹自己;更有甚者表现出自杀、杀人等破坏性的病态反应。

总之,短时间的适当程度的压力能够促进生产力,促进变革。长期的压力可能导致人情绪及行为上的变化,甚至产生身体疾病。

第三节 护士的压力管理

一、护士压力的主要来源

1. 护理患者 繁重的护理工作给护士造成的压力。大部分患者疾病知识缺乏,对医疗技术服务期望过高,认为只要进了医院就没有解决不了的问题。护士应对患者百依百顺,执行治疗、护理操作慢了一点,一针不见血,打针痛了,呼唤帮助不及时,说话语气不注意等都会导致患者的不满意,动不动就对护士发火,甚至投诉、威胁,使护士感觉工作起来太被动,时时处处担惊受怕,很大程度上打击了护士的工作积极性,造成了很大的压力。

2. 工作环境中的压力 医院护理工作平凡、琐碎(如:电灯不亮、暖气不热、空调不凉、患者切口痛、病房陪护多影响患者休息、找不到医生等,他们都会先找护士抱怨);竞争上岗的紧迫感、"三班制"扰乱了护士身体的生活节律;医疗卫生系统中,护士工作辛苦,而报酬相对较低,劳动的付出得不到相应的回报;护士在做各种治疗和护理工作时都在患者、家属,甚至新闻媒体的监督下,这无形中增加了护士的心理压力,易导致心身疾病。此外,护士也面临着一定的职业暴露风险,如:接触艾滋病、梅毒、乙肝等血源性传染病患者。

3. 工作之外的压力 护士的主要性别构成是女性,作为普通职业女性,除了承担职业责任外,还要担负家庭责任和社会责任,既要当好医生的助手、领导和病员的好护士,又要做孝顺的女儿和儿媳、慈爱的母亲、贤惠的妻子,因此工作、社会与家庭都必须兼顾,同时要承担多种角色。这都增加了护士压力。

4. 自我发展受限 随着现代护理学科的发展,护理工作的范围不断扩大,要求护士除了具有高度的责任心、良好的职业道德、较强的临床技能和敏锐的观察力外,还要具有良好的沟通技巧和社会的适应能力。专业的发展,知识结构的更新,各种现代化抢救技术、先进仪器的应用,使护士的自我要求不断提高。但护士继续深造和晋升的机会较少,有相当一部分护士工作一辈子都没有走出本医院学习过,不能与时俱进地掌握新知识、新技术而产生压力。

二、压力管理的方法

1. 培养适应及应对问题的能力 例如:解决问题的技术,批判性的思维方式。认清压力事件的性质,理性思考及分析问题事件的来龙去脉,确认个人对问题的处理能力。运用问题解决技巧,拟定解决计划,积极处理问题。

2. 学习放松技巧

(1)呼吸练习:借由深而长的吸气与呼气,达到放松的效果,一般以腹式呼吸为佳,即吸气时腹部突出,吐气时腹部凹下。

(2)自生训练:基本上是一连串的口语公式,让受试者对自己复述,使自己进入松弛状态,例如:"我感觉很平静、很轻松,我的脚感觉很沉重、很松弛,我的手很重、很温暖"等口语公式。

(3)练气功。

3. 运用好自我防御机制 心理防御机制是人在遭遇挫折时为了抵抗压力,消除恶劣情绪,求得心理平衡的心理自然防御功能。启动心理防御机制的前提是遭遇挫折和应激反应。常见的有否认、幽默、置换、合理化、升华。心理防御机制可以通过多种方式帮助一个人避免或减少焦虑,给对方时间解决可能会让他不知所措的问题,帮助个体学习适应环境的新方法。但心理防御机制只能改变一个人思考和应对压力的方式,不会改变压力情境。

4.养成良好的生活习惯　包括:健康的饮食习惯、充足的睡眠、适度的运动、合理的休息。

5.保持理性　理性做出决策,面对压力冷静理性思考,有效控制情绪。

6.合理规划时间安排　做好时间管理,区分事情的轻重缓急。

7.树立积极正确的人生观　避免过度强调工作或学习,平衡好生活的各个方面,善于思考。

8.完善社会支持系统　和家人、朋友能够诚实地分享自己的问题和情绪,也能给予他人很好的共情。

练习题

1.复杂的亲情关系、子女成长问题、婚姻恋爱关系、家庭发展问题、家庭成员的重大事件等属于(　　)
 A.家庭压力   B.心理压力   C.生理压力   D.社会压力

2.心理压力的机体应对过程不包括(　　)
 A.警戒阶段   B.抵抗阶段   C.疲劳阶段   D.缓和阶段

3.过度的心理压力容易导致的生理症状有(　　)
 A.心跳加速   B.不安   C.易激惹   D.消极怠工

4.过度的心理压力容易导致的心理症状有(　　)
 A.心跳加速   B.呼吸急促   C.人际关系恶化   D.消极怠工

参考答案

参考文献

[1]汪启荣.护理心理学[M].3 版.北京:人民卫生出版社,2020.

[2]陈安娜,陈巍.杜氏反射弧概念中的具身认知思想[J].心理科学,2013,36(1):251-255.

[3]谢弗.发展心健学:儿童与青少年[M].9 版.北京:中国轻工业出版社,2016.

[4]林崇德.学习与发展[M].北京:北京师范大学出版社,1999.

[5]吴昊.家起教育对幼儿心课健康的影响究探究[J].才智,2018,18(25):11-15.

[6]朱智贤.儿童心理学[M].6 版.北京:人民教出版社,2019.

[7]林崇德.发展心理学[M].3 版.北京:人民教育出版社,2018.

[8]黄庭希.当代中国青年价值观与教育[M].成都:四川教育出版社,1994.